RECENT ADVANCES IN HEMATOLOGY RESEARCH

A GUIDE TO PAEDIATRIC RED BLOOD CELL DISORDERS

RECENT ADVANCES IN HEMATOLOGY RESEARCH

Additional books and e-books in this series can be found on Nova's website under the Series tab.

RECENT ADVANCES IN HEMATOLOGY RESEARCH

A GUIDE TO PAEDIATRIC RED BLOOD CELL DISORDERS

SACHITH METTANANDA, MD, DPHIL
DUANTIDA SONGDEJ, MD, DPHIL
AND
THARINDI SURIAPPERUMA, MD

nova
Medicine & Health
New York

Library of Congress Cataloging-in-Publication Data

ISBN: 978-1-53618-695-6
Names: Mettananda, Sachith, author. | Songdej, Duantida, author. | Suriapperuma, Tharindi, author.
Title: A guide to paediatric red blood cell disorder / Sachith Mettananda, University of Kelaniya, Sri Lanka, Duantida Songdej, Tharindi Suriapperuma.
Description: New York : Nova Science Publishers, [2021] | Series: Recent advances in hematology research | Includes bibliographical references and index. |
Identifiers: LCCN 2020043018 (print) | LCCN 2020043019 (ebook) | ISBN 9781536186956 (hardcover) | ISBN 9781536187458 (adobe pdf)
Subjects: LCSH: Erythrocyte disorders--Handbooks, manuals, etc. | Pediatrics--Handbooks, manuals, etc.
Classification: LCC RC647.E7 M48 2021 (print) | LCC RC647.E7 (ebook) | DDC 616.1/51--dc23
LC record available at https://lccn.loc.gov/2020043018
LC ebook record available at https://lccn.loc.gov/2020043019

Published by Nova Science Publishers, Inc. † New York

To children with red blood cell disorders

CONTENTS

FOREWORD

Under the supervision of Sir David Weatherall (FRS) in the 1980s, I became interested in disorders of the Red Cell and I have been particularly focussed on understanding these diseases throughout my life as a clinician and scientist. As the Director of the MRC Weatherall Institute of Molecular Medicine (2012-2020) and Director of the MRC Molecular Haematology Unit (2000-2020), it has been my pleasure to recruit and train many students in how to apply the techniques of molecular biology to problems that arise in clinical medicine and particularly in the management of anaemia. This condition affects 25-30% of the world's population, equivalent to 1.6 billion people, so numerically it is amongst the most important group of disorders affecting human health. Two authors of this book (Sachith Mettananda and Duantida Songdej), which provides a "Guide to Paediatric Red Blood Cell Disorders" were clinical training fellows in my laboratory where they both obtained outstanding DPhils from the University of Oxford. It is also a pleasure to see one's scientific progeny collaborating with other researchers in the same area; in this case the third author is Tharindi Suriapperuma, winner of the Priyani E Soysa Gold Medal for her MD, and currently a colleague of Prof Mettananda at the University of Kelaniya.

These three authors have produced a concise and yet comprehensive book which very nicely covers the topics that arise when considering children with anaemia. It covers the entire range of anaemias one might encounter in paediatric practice: it provides an excellent guide to the uninitiated and a perfect aide memoire for those already familiar with these conditions. It covers the approach to thinking about this group of disorders, their classification, their pathophysiology, including their molecular basis when known, and the best approaches to their diagnosis and treatment. This short book is not meant to be a definitive textbook rather it is a very helpful guide to what can be a bewildering set of disorders. For those wishing to have more detailed understanding the authors have provided some key references at the end of each section for further reading.

I can thoroughly recommend this book to clinicians at all stages of their careers whether medical students, registrars or consultants wishing to refresh their understanding of childhood anaemia. The book is also useful for researchers wishing to rapidly grasp an overview of this area of clinical medicine as part of new scientific projects and programmes. It can be read in a short time as a review or kept on the shelf to dip into as questions arise. Having read through this very nice book, I will certainly be keeping it close to hand for frequent future reference.

Professor Doug Higgs, FMedSci FRS
Emeritus Professor of Haematology
Former Director (2012-2020)
MRC Weatherall Institute of Molecular Medicine
University of Oxford, United Kingdom
August 2020

PREFACE

A Guide to Paediatric Red Blood Cell Disorders aims to provide comprehensive and up-to-date information on common red blood cell diseases encountered in children. Here, we cover the entire breadth from molecular pathology to the current treatment of most paediatric red cell disorders. This book is intended to be a useful guide to postgraduate doctors training in paediatrics and haematology, medical undergraduates, primary care physicians and practising clinicians.

The book is divided into five sections. The first section, which is on basic concepts and an approach to red blood cell disorders in children, provides information on the structure and function of red blood cells and haemoglobin, epidemiology and aetiology of anaemia and clinical and laboratory evaluation of a child with anaemia. This section is particularly useful for undergraduate and postgraduate students who are preparing for their clinical examinations as well as for practising clinicians. The next three sections will provide information on paediatric conditions that result in microcytic, normocytic and macrocytic anaemia, respectively. The final section will be on conditions leading to polycythaemia in neonates and children.

Throughout the book, the emphasis has been given to common conditions that are frequently encountered in clinical practice. However, rare but clinically important conditions have also been included. Each chapter is divided into subsections to cover the epidemiology, aetiology, genetic basis, molecular pathology, pathophysiology, classification, clinical features, investigations, diagnosis, treatment, follow-up and prognosis of each disorder. At the end of each chapter, a section on recent advances will provide information on promising novel developments and experimental approaches for treating these diseases.

We have taken every possible step to provide the most up-to-date information on all aspects of diseases. The book is concise, reader-friendly and written in simple English, which could be understood by non-native speakers. We hope that this book will be a useful guide to readers across the world who are managing red blood cell disorders of children.

Sachith Mettananda
Duantida Songdej
Tharindi Suriapperuma
August 2020

LIST OF ABBREVIATIONS

ACE	Angiotensin converting enzyme
aHUS	Atypical haemolytic uremic syndrome
AIHA	Autoimmune haemolytic anaemia
AML	Acute myeloid leukaemia
APTT	Activated partial thromboplastin time
ATP	Adenosine triphosphate
CAD	Cold agglutinin disease
CDA	Congenital dyserythropoietic anaemia
CSA	Congenital sideroblastic anaemia
DAT	Direct antiglobulin test
DBA	Diamond Blackfan anaemia
DIC	Disseminated intravascular coagulation
DNA	Deoxyribonucleic acid
eADA	Erythrocyte adenosine deaminase activity
EMA	Eosin-5-maleimide
FDP	Fibrinogen degradation products
G6PD	Glucose 6-phosphate dehydrogenase
HbA	Haemoglobin A / Adult haemoglobin
HbA_2	Haemoglobin A_2
HbE	Haemoglobin E
HbF	Haemoglobin F / Fetal haemoglobin
HbH	Haemoglobin H

HDFN	Haemolytic disease of the fetus and newborn
HLA	Human leukocyte antigen
HPLC	High performance liquid chromatography
HSC	Haematopoietic stem cell
HUS	Haemolytic uremic syndrome
IAT	Indirect antiglobulin test
IDA	Iron deficiency anaemia
IgA	Imunoglobulin A
IgG	Imunoglobulin G
IgM	Imunoglobulin M
IRIDA	Iron refractory iron deficiency anaemia
KMP	Kasabach-Merritt phenomenon
MAHA	Microangiopathic haemolytic anaemia
MCH	Mean corpuscular haemoglobin
MCHC	Mean corpuscular haemoglobin concentration
MCV	Mean corpuscular volume
MDS	Myelodysplastic syndrome
MRA	Magnetic resonance angiogram
MRI	Magnetic resonance imaging
NADP	Nicotinamide adenine dinucleotide phosphate
PCH	Paroxysmal cold haemoglobinuria
PCR	Polymerase chain reaction
PNH	Paroxysmal nocturnal haemoglobinuria
RBC	Red blood cell
RDW	Red cell distribution width
RNA	Ribonucleic acid
SCA	Sickle cell anaemia
SCD	Sickle cell disease
STEC	Shiga toxin-producing *Escherichia coli*
TEC	Transient erythroblastopenia of childhood
TMA	Thrombotic microangiopathy
TTP	Thrombotic thrombocytopenic purpura
WHO	World Health Organization

Part 1.
Basic Concepts and an Approach to Red Blood Cell Disorders

Chapter 1

Red Blood Cells and Haemoglobin

Sachith Mettananda*

Department of Paediatrics, University of Kelaniya, Ragama, Sri Lanka

Red Blood Cells

Red blood cell (RBC) is the most abundant blood cell of humans. Mature RBCs which are also referred to as erythrocytes have a diameter of approximately 7-8μm. These flexible, oval, biconcave cells do not contain a cell nucleus or organelles. Most of the cytoplasm is filled with haemoglobin which is the primary oxygen-carrying molecule of humans.

RBCs are produced following a series of cell division and differentiation steps from haematopoietic stem cells (HSC) through a process known as erythropoiesis. During erythropoiesis, multipotent HSCs which reside in the bone marrow differentiate through various progenitor stages to the earliest morphologically identifiable erythroid precursors, proerythroblasts. Thereafter, during terminal differentiation, proerythro-

* Corresponding Author's Email: sachith.mettananda@kln.ac.lk.

blasts become progressively smaller and undergo nuclear condensation to differentiate into basophilic, polychromatophilic and orthochromatic erythroblasts which then enucleate to form reticulocytes and mature RBCs.

Throughout embryonic and fetal development, the site of erythropoiesis changes. During the early embryonic period, a transient cohort of embryonic RBCs originates in the blood islands of the yolk sac. Definitive HSCs then emerge from the ventral wall of the dorsal aorta which migrate to the fetal liver midway in the first trimester. Around the time of birth, HSCs migrate to the bone marrow, which is the principal site of erythropoiesis for the rest of the life.

A normal healthy human adult produces approximately two million RBCs per second in the bone marrow. The average life span of a RBC is 100 to 120 days. During its lifespan, a human RBC travels approximately 500km, making nearly 170,000 circuits through the heart. The primary physiological role of RBCs is to transport O_2 from lungs to the tissues and CO_2 from tissues to the lungs. For effective functioning, RBCs have a number of adaptations; they contain a large amount of haemoglobin that can reversibly bind to oxygen; they are small, flexible and highly deformable cells that can traverse through blood vessels as narrow as 3-4μm; and they are biconcave cells thus have maximum surface area for a unit volume to allow efficient diffusion of gases.

STRUCTURE OF HAEMOGLOBIN

Haemoglobin is the oxygen-carrying molecule of the human body. It is a 64-kD protein composed of four globin peptide chains, each of which are associated with a haem moiety. Four globin chains of a haemoglobin molecule are arranged as heterodimers of two α-like and two β-like globin chains. The haem moiety which is linked to a histidine residue of each globin subunit is formed by a single molecule of protoporphyrin IX bound to a ferrous (Fe^{++}) ion. In the ferrous form, the haem group can bind to gaseous ligands, including O_2.

Globin genes are the most extensively studied and characterized gene loci in the human genome. The α- and β-globin gene loci are located in two different chromosomes. The human α-globin gene cluster is located on the short arm of chromosome 16 (16p13.3) close (~150kb) to the telomere. In this 135kb segment, globin genes are arranged in the order in which they are expressed during development; telomere-ζ-μ-α_2-α_1-centromere (Figure 1.1). Similarly, several β-like globin genes are located in the order of their expression during development in the human β-globin gene locus in chromosome 11 (11p). The arrangement of genes in this locus is, telomere-ε-$^G\gamma$-$^A\gamma$-δ-β-centromere.

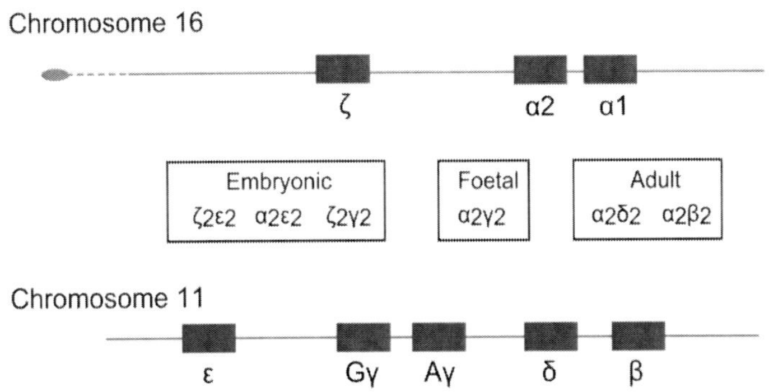

Figure 1.1. A schematic diagram of α- and β-globin gene clusters and the types of haemoglobin produced at each developmental stage. Genes are arranged along the chromosome in the order in which they are expressed during development: in the α-cluster ζ (embryonic) and α (embryonic, fetal, and adult); in the β-cluster ε (embryonic), γ (fetal), and δ and β (adult).

The expression of globin genes shows a well-coordinated and developmental-stage-specific expression pattern throughout development. At the α-globin locus, both ζ- and α-globin genes are expressed during the embryonic period. However, the ζ-globin genes are silenced during fetal and postnatal stages. In the β-globin locus, ε- and γ-globin is expressed during embryonic and fetal periods respectively, and then γ-globin is switched to β-globin (and to a lesser extent δ-globin) after birth (Figure 1.2). These changes are associated with changes in the types of haemoglobin produced. Haemoglobin Gower-I ($\zeta_2\varepsilon_2$), haemoglobin Gower-

II ($\alpha_2\varepsilon_2$) and haemoglobin Portland ($\zeta_2\gamma_2$) are produced during the embryonic stages which are then switched, first, to haemoglobin F (HbF, $\alpha_2\gamma_2$) during the fetal stage and subsequently, to haemoglobin A (HbA, $\alpha_2\beta_2$) and A_2 (HbA_2, $\alpha_2\delta_2$) after birth.

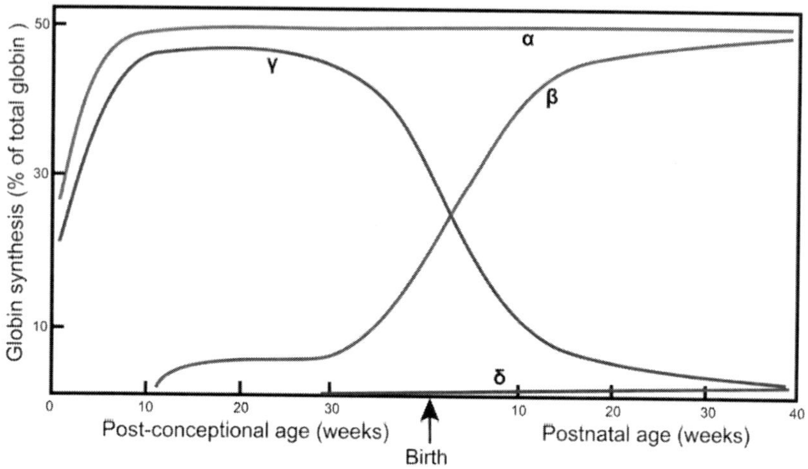

Figure 1.2. Developmental expression of the human globin genes. ζ and ε are the first globin genes to be expressed during the embryonic stage (not shown) and are then switched to α and γ in the foetal stage. The second globin switch from γ to β occurs during the first few months after birth.

FUNCTIONS OF HAEMOGLOBIN

The primary function of haemoglobin is to transport oxygen from the lungs to the tissues. Haemoglobin forms a dissociable complex with oxygen. Each deoxyhaemoglobin molecule can reversibly bind to four ions of oxygen in the presence of high oxygen partial pressures as in lungs to form oxyhaemoglobin which can release oxygen in situations of low oxygen partial pressures as in tissues. Oxygenation of haemoglobin as a function of the oxygen concentration is expressed by a sigmoid oxy-haemoglobin dissociation curve.

Oxygen affinity of haemoglobin is designated by the P_{50}, which is the partial pressure of oxygen at which haemoglobin is 50% saturated. The P_{50}

of HbA is 27 mmHg at 37°C and a pH of 7.4. High temperature, acidosis and higher 2,3-bisphosphoglycerate levels decrease the oxygen affinity and thus cause a right shift of the oxy-haemoglobin dissociation curve. Conversely, decreasing temperature, alkalosis and lower 2,3-bisphosphoglycerate increase the oxygen affinity of haemoglobin and result in a left shift of the oxy-haemoglobin dissociation curve. Also, HbF has a higher affinity for oxygen compared to HbA.

Disorders of Red Blood Cells

RBC disorders are of two main forms. Conditions that lead to a decrease in RBCs and haemoglobin are known as anaemia, whereas conditions that result in abnormal excess of RBCs are known as polycythaemia. In children, anaemia is by far the most prevalent clinical condition.

References

Gell, D. A. 2018. "Structure and function of haemoglobins." *Blood Cells Mol Dis* 70:13-42. doi: 10.1016/j.bcmd.2017.10.006.

Higgs, DR, N Roy, and D Hay. 2015. "Erythropoiesis." In *Postgraduate Haematology*, edited by AV Hoffbrand, DR Higgs, DM Keeling and AB Mehta, 11-21. NJ: Wiley-Blackwell.

Kuhn, V., L. Diederich, T. C. S. th Keller, C. M. Kramer, W. Lückstädt, C. Panknin, T. Suvorava, B. E. Isakson, M. Kelm, and M. M. Cortese-Krott. 2017. "Red Blood Cell Function and Dysfunction: Redox Regulation, Nitric Oxide Metabolism, Anemia." *Antioxid Redox Signal* 26 (13):718-742. doi: 10.1089/ars.2016.6954.

Mettananda, S., and D. R. Higgs. 2018. "Molecular Basis and Genetic Modifiers of Thalassemia." *Hematol Oncol Clin North Am* 32 (2):177-191. doi: 10.1016/j.hoc.2017.11.003.

Sankaran, V. G., and M. J. Weiss. 2015. "Anemia: progress in molecular mechanisms and therapies." *Nat Med* 21 (3):221-30. doi: 10.1038/nm.3814.

Steinberg, Martin H., Bernard G. Forget, Douglas R. Higgs, and David J. Weatherall. 2009. *Disorders of Hemoglobin: Genetics, Pathophysiology, and Clinical Management*. 2nd ed, *Cambridge Medicine*. Cambridge: Cambridge University Press.

Weatherall, D. J., and J. B. Clegg. 2001. *The thalassaemia syndromes*. 4 ed. Oxford: Blackwell Science.

Chapter 2

EVALUATION OF CHILDHOOD ANAEMIA

Sachith Mettananda*
Department of Paediatrics, University of Kelaniya, Ragama, Sri Lanka

DEFINITION OF ANAEMIA

Anaemia is defined as having lower than normal red blood cell (RBC) mass or haemoglobin concentration for the age, sex and physiological state. The cut-off values of haemoglobin to diagnose anaemia in children do not have consensus agreement; however, the values advocated by the World Health Organisation are generally accepted worldwide (Table 2.1). The highest levels of haemoglobin at any age is observed soon after birth. In the newborn, the normal haemoglobin level is 15-24g/dL. Thereafter, the haemoglobin drops rapidly during the first few weeks of life to a nadir of 9-10g/dL around two months of age. Subsequently, haemoglobin gradually rises and stabilises above 11g/dL by the age of six months. Therefore, haemoglobin level below 11g/dL in a child aged between six

* Corresponding Author's Email: sachith.mettananda@kln.ac.lk.

months to five years or below 11.5g/dL in a child aged between 5-12 years is considered as anaemia.

Table 2.1. Cut-off haemoglobin values to diagnose anaemia in children

	Cut-off value to diagnose anaemia (g/dL)	Severity of anaemia (g/dL)		
		Mild	Moderate	Severe
Neonate	<15.0			
6 months – 4 years	<11.0	10.0 – 10.9	7.0 – 9.9	<7.0
5 – 11 years	<11.5	11.0 – 11.4	8.0 – 10.9	<8.0
12 – 14years	<12.0	11.0 – 11.9	8.0 – 10.9	<8.0

EPIDEMIOLOGY

Anaemia is one of the most common public health problems in the world. It is estimated that approximately 25-30% of the world population or 1.6 billion people across the globe suffer from anaemia. The prevalence of anaemia is high among certain risk populations. Children less than five years, females in the childbearing age, pregnant females and elderly are more prone to develop anaemia than others. The global prevalence of anaemia among preschool and school-going children is reported as 47% and 25% respectively. The highest prevalence of childhood anaemia is reported in Africa (67%) and South Asia (65%) whereas Europe (21%) has the lowest prevalence.

AETIOLOGICAL CLASSIFICATION

The aetiology of anaemia in children is diverse. The causes of anaemia can be classified based on the RBC size or mechanism of causation. Based on the RBC size, anaemia is classified into microcytic, normocytic and macrocytic anaemia. Classification based on the mechanism divides causes of anaemia into two main groups; anaemia due to reduced production and anaemia due to increased loss (Figure 2.1).

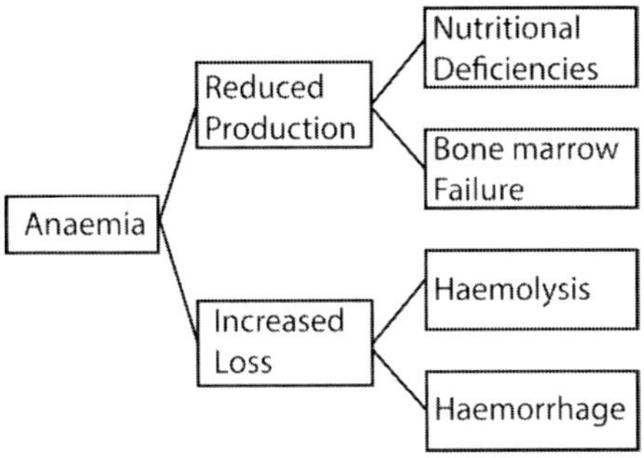

Figure 2.1. Classification of mechanisms causing anaemia.

Decreased production of RBCs could be due to two reasons. Firstly, it can result from deficiencies of micronutrients that are essential for RBC synthesis. These nutrients are iron, folate and vitamin B12. Secondly, it can be due to pathology of the bone marrow caused by bone marrow failure or infiltration.

Increased loss of RBCs is either due to haemolysis or haemorrhage; of these haemolytic anaemias are the most important group. Causes of haemolytic anaemia are subdivided into two main categories; haemolysis due to intrinsic defects of the RBCs or extrinsic factors. Intrinsic defects of RBCs are mostly due to inherited genetic diseases which are further divided into three types. Firstly, abnormalities in erythroid membrane proteins, for example, hereditary spherocytosis and hereditary elliptocytosis are known as membranopathies. Secondly, mutations in the critical RBC enzymes such as glucose 6-phosphate dehydrogenase (G6PD) and pyruvate kinase are called enzymopathies. Thirdly, defective synthesis of haemoglobin due to thalassaemia or structural defects are labelled as haemoglobinopathies. Examples for extrinsic factors causing haemolysis are immune-mediated haemolysis, drugs, toxins and mechanical destruction of erythrocytes (Table 2.2).

Another classification categorises haemolytic anaemias based on the site of RBC destruction. Haemolysis that occur outside blood vessels, usually within phagocytic macrophages in the spleen, liver or lymph nodes is named extravascular haemolysis. Hereditary spherocytosis, hereditary elliptocytosis, pyruvate kinase deficiency and warm type autoimmune haemolytic anaemia (AIHA) are examples for this type of haemolysis. Conversely, haemolysis occurring within blood vessels while in the circulation is termed intravascular haemolysis. G6PD deficiency, cold type AIHA and microangiopathic haemolytic anaemia (MAHA) are examples for intravascular haemolysis.

Table 2.2. Aetiology of childhood anaemia

- **Anaemia due to reduced production of RBCs**
  - *Nutritional deficiencies*
    - Iron deficiency
    - Folic acid deficiency
    - Vitamin B12 deficiency
  - *Bone marrow failure or infiltration*
    - Pure red cell aplasia (e.g., Diamond Blackfan Anaemia, Transient erythroblastopenia of childhood, Red cell aplasia associated with parvovirus B19 infection)
    - Aplastic anaemia (e.g., Fanconi anaemia, Acquired aplastic anaemia)
    - Haematological malignancies (e.g., Acute leukaemia, Lymphoma)
    - Anaemia of chronic disease
- **Anaemia due to increased loss of RBCs**
  - *Haemolytic anaemia*
    - *Membranopathies*
      - Hereditary spherocytosis
      - Hereditary elliptocytosis
    - *Enzymopathies*
      - Glucose 6-phosphate dehydrogenase deficiency
      - Pyruvate kinase deficiency
    - *Haemoglobin disorders*
      - Thalassaemia (e.g., β-thalassaemia, α-thalassaemia, HbE disease)
      - Sickle cell disease
      - Other haemoglobinopathies
    - *Extracellular factors*
      - Autoimmune haemolytic anaemia
      - Haemolytic uremic syndrome
      - Thrombotic thrombocytopenic purpura
      - Disseminated intravascular coagulation
      - Drugs and toxins
      - Haemangiomas
  - *Haemorrhage*

CLINICAL EVALUATION – HISTORY

A vast majority of children with anaemia are asymptomatic; therefore, are diagnosed during physical examination or investigations performed for different reasons. In both symptomatic and asymptomatic patients, a careful evaluation with a detailed history and a complete physical examination followed by stepwise investigations is essential to narrow down the differential diagnosis of anaemia. The important aspects in the clinical history of a patient with anaemia are described below.

Symptoms of Anaemia

Common symptoms of anaemia reported by children include lethargy, irritability, poor feeding and exercise intolerance. These symptoms are present only in patients who have severe anaemia or anaemia which is of rapid onset.

Onset and Duration of Anaemia

The duration of anaemia provides useful information to identify its cause. Most pathologies that cause anaemia has an insidious onset. However, acute-onset anaemia is seen in G6PD deficiency, bone marrow infiltration such as in acute leukaemia, AIHA and MAHA that includes haemolytic uremic syndrome (HUS), thrombotic thrombocytopenic purpura (TTP) and disseminated intravascular coagulation (DIC).

Bleeding Manifestations

Both revealed and concealed bleeding could lead to anaemia. Noteworthy bleeding from the gastrointestinal tract manifesting as melena or per rectal bleeding could result in anaemia due to direct blood loss. Conversely, prolonged minor bleeds can result in iron deficiency anaemia (IDA). Alternatively, bleeding can be a symptom of thrombocytopenia which is associated with anaemia in bone marrow pathologies.

Urine Colour

Dark red or cola colour urine suggests haemoglobinuria due to intravascular haemolysis in haemolytic anaemias. Dark colour urine is also seen in haemolytic anaemia due to high levels of bilirubin in urine.

Past History

The history of previous episodes of anaemia should be obtained from all patients. A careful review of previous haemoglobin values and RBC indices would provide useful information on the chronicity of anaemia. Additionally, a history of underlying medical conditions or chronic diseases may indicate anaemia of chronic disease.

Birth History

Babies who are born prematurely can develop anaemia of prematurity during the first few months of life. History of hyperbilirubinemia requiring phototherapy or exchange transfusion during the neonatal period is suggestive of a haemolytic disease like hereditary spherocytosis, G6PD deficiency or pyruvate kinase deficiency.

Developmental History

Children with Fanconi anaemia and Diamond Blackfan anaemia (DBA) can have associated global developmental delay. Therefore, a detailed development history is vital if these diseases are suspected.

Dietary History

Several micronutrient deficiencies, especially deficiencies of iron, folate and vitamin B12 are common causes for anaemia in children. Dietary history should focus on the adequacy of diets rich in these micronutrients as well as macronutrients.

Drug History

A number of drugs including antibiotics, antimalarials and analgesics, can precipitate haemolysis in G6PD deficiency (see table 8.2 for the full list of drugs). Therefore, it is important to inquire about drug history, especially in patients with acute-onset anaemia.

Family History

Several haematological conditions causing anaemia are genetically inherited diseases. Hereditary spherocytosis is autosomal dominant, thalassaemia and sickle cell disease are autosomal recessive and G6PD deficiency is X-linked. A family history of anaemia or splenomegaly can indicate any of these diseases. Also, parental consanguinity increases the risk of autosomal recessive disorders like thalassaemia and sickle cell disease.

Social History

Malaria is a well-recognised cause of anaemia in children. Therefore, a recent travel history to tropical African regions or India, which has a high prevalence of malaria points towards infective causes of anaemia.

Clinical Evaluation – Examination

Aims of physical examination of children with anaemia are to identify the aetiology and to look for complications related to anaemia and specific diagnoses. The examination should focus on the following;

General Appearance

The general appearance of a child could provide valuable information regarding the cause of anaemia. Most children with mild to moderate anaemia would appear well. Irritability, excessive crying and listlessness are general examination findings of anaemia.

Pallor

Conjunctival and skin pallor provides a rough assessment of the degree of anaemia. As pallor is clinically detectable only when the haemoglobin drops below 8-9g/dL, a majority of asymptomatic children with anaemia may not be pale.

Jaundice

Jaundice or yellowish discolouration of body and sclerae occur due to increased unconjugated bilirubin. It is indicative of haemolytic anaemia.

Growth Parameters

Growth can get affected by severe anaemia. Conversely, some causes of anaemia (e.g., Fanconi anaemia) are associated with short stature.

Facial Appearance

Bone marrow expansion due to excessive erythropoiesis leads to disfiguring facial appearance. The specific signs are frontal bossing, maxillary hyperplasia and dental malocclusion. These features suggest chronic severe haemolytic process like thalassaemia major. Due to early diagnosis and improved management, these manifestations are rare at present except in extreme cases.

Skin Manifestations

Hyperpigmentation and café-au-lait patches are associated with Fanconi anaemia. Petechiae and purpura are suggestive of mucocutaneous bleeding due to thrombocytopenia or bone marrow infiltration. The skin due to nutritional deficiency can be coarse and rough to the touch.

Thumb Abnormalities

Abnormalities in thumbs are recognised clinical features of Fanconi anaemia.

Nutritional Deficiencies

Angular stomatitis, glossitis and koilonychia are physical signs that are seen in children with severe iron deficiency. Presence of these in a child with anaemia suggest iron deficiency as the possible cause.

Hepatomegaly

Hepatomegaly in children with anaemia is suggestive of thalassaemia or haematological malignancies. In thalassaemia, hepatomegaly is the result of extramedullary haematopoiesis, whereas in haematological malignancies it results from leukaemic infiltration.

Splenomegaly

In patients with anaemia, the presence of splenomegaly suggests thalassaemia, haematological malignancies or conditions associated with extravascular haemolysis (e.g., hereditary spherocytosis and elliptocytosis). Membranopathies like hereditary spherocytosis causes mild splenomegaly, whereas thalassaemia can cause splenomegaly of any size.

Lymphadenopathy

Generalised lymphadenopathy in a child with anaemia is highly suggestive of haematological malignancies.

Initial Investigation – Full Blood Count

Full blood count report from an automated analyser will aid to narrow down the differential diagnosis of anaemia substantially. Following useful information can be obtained from a full blood count report;

Haemoglobin

The haemoglobin level is essential to confirm anaemia as well as to determine the severity of anaemia.

Mean Corpuscular Volume

Mean corpuscular volume (MCV), which measures the size of RBCs, is possibly the next most crucial parameter in a full blood count. The normal range of MCV varies with age (Table 2.3). However, in general, a range of 75-95fL is considered normal for children. Based on the MCV, anaemia is classified into three types; microcytic anaemia (small RBCs; MCV<75fL), normocytic anaemia (normal size RBCs; MCV 75-95fL) and macrocytic anaemia (larger RBCs; MCV>95fl).

Mean Corpuscular Haemoglobin

Mean corpuscular haemoglobin (MCH) is a measure of haemoglobin content in a RBC. The normal range of MCH is also dependent on age (Table 2.3). A low MCH indicates decreased haemoglobin content per cell and is typically seen in iron deficiency and thalassaemia.

Table 2.3. Normal values of red blood cell indices at different ages

	Normal range for MCV (fL)	Normal range for MCH (pg)	Normal range for MCHC (g/dL)
1 – 30 days	99 – 115	33 – 39	32 – 36
1 – 23 months	72 – 88	24 – 30	32 – 36
2 – 9 years	76 – 90	25 – 31	32 – 36
10 – 16 years	78 – 95	26 – 32	32 – 36

Mean Corpuscular Haemoglobin Concentration

Low mean corpuscular haemoglobin concentration (MCHC) is typical of iron deficiency, and high MCHC values are suggestive of the presence of spherocytes.

Red Cell Distribution Width

The red cell distribution width (RDW) is a measure of the variation in RBC size. A high RDW implies a considerable variation in RBC size, whereas a low RDW implies a homogeneous population of RBCs. High RDW is characteristic of IDA.

Reticulocyte Count and Percentage

Normal reticulocyte percentage is 1-2%. Reticulocytosis (>2%) suggests haemolytic anaemia while reticulocytopenia is suggestive of RBC aplasia or aplastic anaemia.

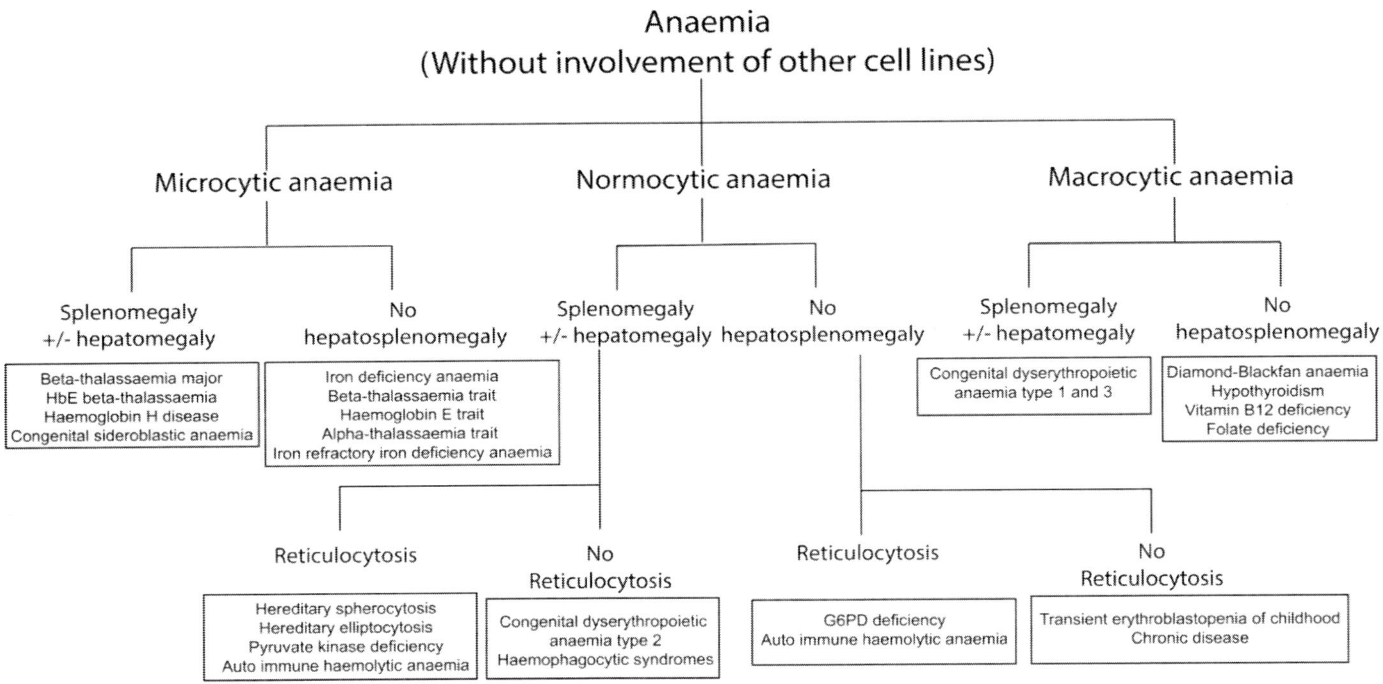

Figure 2.2. An approach to narrow down the differential diagnosis in a child presenting with anaemia without abnormalities in the white blood cells and platelets.

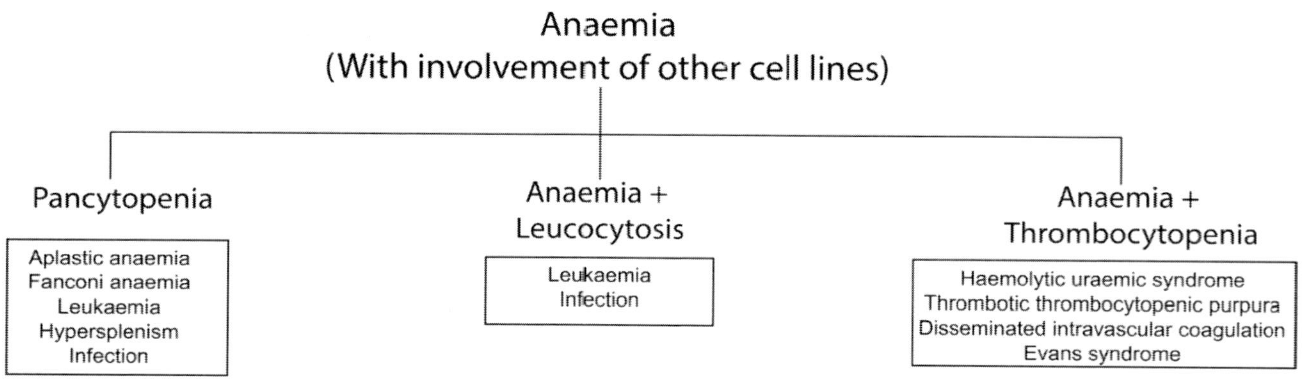

Figure 2.3. An approach to identifying the aetiology in children who present with anaemia with abnormalities in white blood cells or platelets.

White Blood Cell Count

White blood cell count provides useful information on the involvement of other cell lines in the haematopoietic lineage. Leukopenia suggests bone marrow failure or hypersplenism and leucocytosis support a diagnosis of haematological malignancy. However, normal white blood cell count does not exclude leukaemia.

Platelet Count

Bicytopenia due to anaemia and thrombocytopenia is suggestive of either MAHA or immune-mediated destruction of both RBCs and platelets due to Evans syndrome. Also, it can be a part of pancytopenia due to hypersplenism, bone marrow failure or infiltration into the bone marrow.

Based on the clinical findings and results of full blood count, differential diagnosis of anaemia in children can be narrowed down to a considerable extent. Figure 2.2 presents a rational guide to arrive at a diagnosis when anaemia is isolated without the involvement of other cell lines (white blood cells and platelets). Figure 2.3 provides the differential diagnosis when anaemia is associated with abnormalities in other cell lines. Further confirmatory investigations should be based on the likely diagnosis according to these flowcharts.

Investigations of Microcytic Anaemia

Microcytic anaemia is the most common type of anaemia seen in children. IDA and haemoglobinopathies like thalassaemia are important differential diagnoses for microcytic anaemia in children. The most helpful investigations in differentiating these two conditions are serum ferritin and haemoglobin subtype quantification by high-performance liquid chromate-graphy (HPLC) or capillary electrophoresis.

Blood Film

Blood film will confirm the presence of microcytic hypochromic RBCs (Figure 2.4). The presence of pencil-shaped cells, teardrop cells and anisopoikilocytosis suggest iron deficiency whereas target cells and nucleated RBCs suggest haemoglobinopathy.

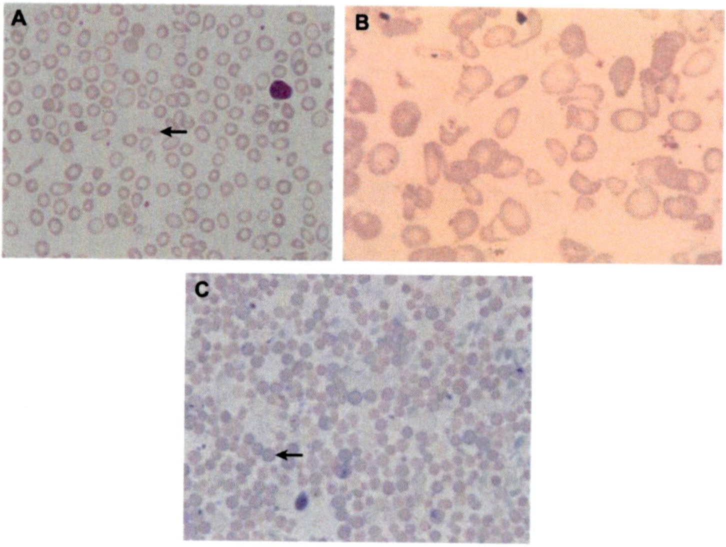

Figure 2.4. Blood film characteristics of microcytic anaemia. (A) Blood film of IDA showing microcytic hypochromic RBCs and pencil shaped cells (arrow). (B) Blood film of β-thalassaemia showing anisopoikilocytosis. (C) Haemoglobin H inclusion bodies (arrow) in haemoglobin H disease.

Serum Ferritin

Serum ferritin is the most widely used investigation to diagnose iron deficiency. Although the reference range may vary from laboratory to laboratory, a serum ferritin value less than 15ng/mL in a child is confirmatory of IDA. However, serum ferritin is an acute-phase protein thus, can erroneously be elevated in the presence of inflammation leading to falsely high values.

Serum Iron Profile

Iron profile includes, serum iron, total iron-binding capacity and percentage saturation of transferrin. Serum iron profile is less affected by inflammation; therefore, it is suitable in a child with infection or inflammation. In iron deficiency, serum iron is low, total iron-binding capacity is increased, and transferrin saturation is <16%.

Haemoglobin Subtype Quantification

Haemoglobin subtype quantification by HPLC or capillary electrophoresis is useful in diagnosing β-haemoglobinopathies (Table 2.4). In instances where interpretation is difficult, family screening with HPLC or capillary electrophoresis studies of parents and siblings are helpful.

Table 2.4. Quantification of haemoglobin subtypes in haemoglobinopathies

	HbA	HbA_2	HbF	Other
Normal	>95%	<3.4%	<2%	-
β-Thalassaemia trait	>90%	3.5%-7.0%	1-3%	-
HbE trait	50-80%	<3.4%	1-3%	HbE: 20-50%
HbS trait	50-70%	<3.4%	1-3%	HbS: 20-40%
β-Thalassaemia major	<10%	2-5%	>70%	-
HbE β-thalassaemia	<10%	<3.4%	30%-70%	HbE: 30%-50%
HbS β-thalassaemia	<30%	<7.0%	<20%	HbS: 50%-80%
Sickle cell anaemia	0	<3.4%	5%-15%	HbS: 80%-95%
α-Thalassaemia	>90%	<3.4%	<2%	-

Normal serum ferritin or iron profile and normal haemoglobin subtype quantification exclude both iron deficiency and β-haemoglobinopathy in a child with microcytic anaemia. Among such children, a vast majority have α-thalassaemia trait. Similarly, iron deficiency can coexist with α- or β-thalassaemia. Therefore, it is essential to investigate for β-thalassaemia trait even if a diagnosis of iron deficiency is made in a child with microcytic anaemia.

α-Globin Gene Molecular Studies

α-Thalassaemia trait could only be diagnosed by molecular studies. Several deletional α-thalassaemia mutations can be identified by multiplexed polymerase chain reaction method.

Haemoglobin H inclusion Bodies

Haemoglobin H is an abnormal haemoglobin tetramer composed of four β-globin chains (β_4). The presence of haemoglobin H inclusion bodies in the supravital staining of peripheral blood film is indicative of haemoglobin H disease, which is a subtype of α-thalassaemia (Figure 2.4).

Bone Marrow Aspiration and Biopsy

Bone marrow aspiration and biopsy are rarely required in the investigation of hypochromic microcytic anaemia. The only indication is in a child with microcytic anaemia and hepatosplenomegaly in whom thalassaemia is conclusively excluded. These children could have rare congenital sideroblastic anaemia which is diagnosed by the presence of ring sideroblasts in the bone marrow.

Genetic Studies to Identify Mutations Causing Iron Refractory Iron Deficiency Anaemia

Iron refractory iron deficiency anaemia is suspected in children who have identical clinical and laboratory characteristics of IDA (microcytic anaemia and low serum ferritin) but do not respond to oral iron. This rare entity is due to a variety of genetic mutations of which mutations in the *TMPRSS6* gene are well characterized. These mutations can be identified by DNA sequencing.

Investigations of Normocytic Anaemia

Normocytic anaemia is most commonly due to haemolytic anaemia or bone marrow failure. It may or may not be associated with involvement of other cell lines. Following investigations aid to arrive at the diagnosis when normocytic anaemia is not associated with abnormalities in white blood cells or platelets.

Reticulocyte Count

Reticulocytes are immature erythroid cells which retain their ribosomal network that is stained with supravital stains. Reticulocytosis (reticulocyte count >2%) is indicative of haemolytic anaemia while reticulocytopenia is an indicator of bone marrow aplasia.

Blood Film

Blood film is possibly the most useful investigation to find the cause in a child with normocytic anaemia. Most haemolytic anaemias have characteristic blood film features that include;

- Microspherocytes – hereditary spherocytosis or AIHA;
- Elliptocytes – hereditary elliptocytosis;
- Bite cells and blister cells – G6PD deficiency;
- Fragmented red blood cells (schistocytes and helmet cells) – MAHA.

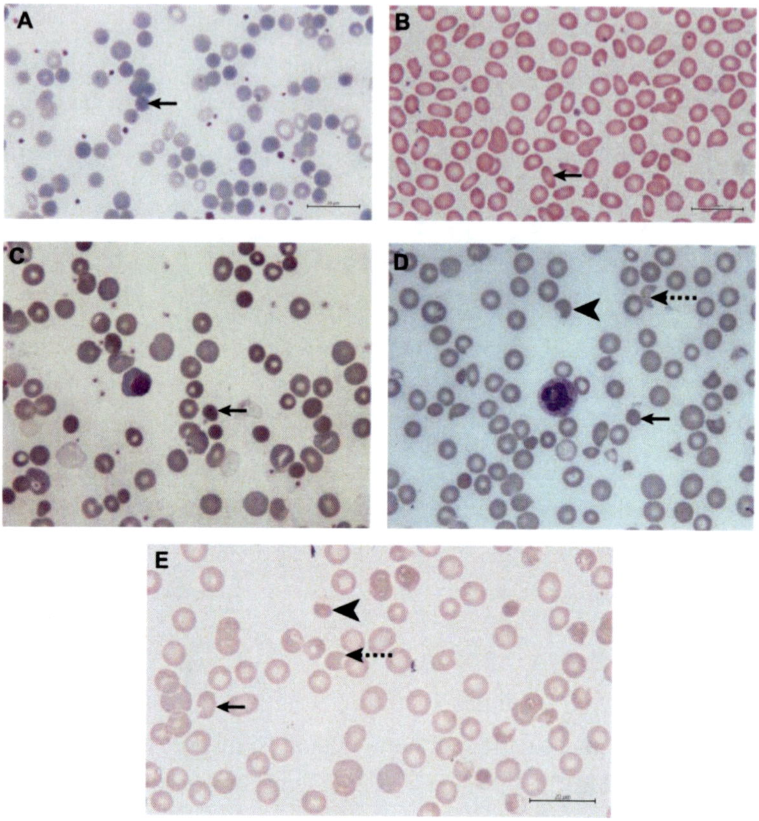

Figure 2.5. Blood film characteristics of normocytic anaemia. (A) Blood film of hereditary spherocytosis showing microspherocytes (arrow). (B) Blood film of hereditary elliptocytosis showing elliptocytes (arrow). (C) Blood film of autoimmune haemolytic anaemia showing microspherocytes (arrow). (D) Blood film of microangiopathic haemolytic anaemia showing schistocytes (arrowhead), fragmented cells (dashed arrow) and microspherocytes (arrow). (E) Blood film of G6PD deficiency showing bite cells (arrow), blister cells (dashed arrow) and contracted haemoglobin RBCs (arrowhead).

Additionally, blood film will be useful in evaluating abnormalities in white blood cells (e.g., blast cells in acute leukaemia) and platelets (e.g., thrombocytopenia in MAHA and large platelets in Evans syndrome) that points towards a diagnosis in normocytic anaemia.

Serum Bilirubin

Breakdown in haem present in haemoglobin leads to the formation of bilirubin. Therefore, haemolytic anaemias result in an increase in the serum levels of unconjugated bilirubin which is reported as an indirect fraction of bilirubin.

Serum Lactate Dehydrogenase

Lactate dehydrogenase is a cytoplasmic enzyme present in many tissues, including erythrocytes. Although non-specific, elevated levels of serum lactate dehydrogenase in a child with anaemia suggests a haemolytic process.

Haemoglobinuria

Presence of haemoglobin will make urine dark red or cola colour. Haemoglobinuria is an indicator of intravascular haemolysis.

Direct Agglutination Test

Positive direct agglutination test (Direct Coombs test) is suggestive of immune-mediated haemolysis and AIHA.

Osmotic Fragility Test

Osmotic fragility is increased in the presence of spherocytes in hereditary spherocytosis. However, this test is not specific for hereditary spherocytosis. It may be positive in the presence of autoimmune haemolysis as well in the presence of microspherocytes. Cryohaemolysis test and acidified glycerol lysis test are alternatives for osmotic fragility test.

G6PD Enzyme Activity

Decreased G6PD enzyme activity in red blood cells is confirmatory of G6PD deficiency. However, this test can be falsely negative during a haemolytic crisis of G6PD deficiency. To confirm G6PD deficiency, G6PD enzyme levels should be repeated approximately 3-4 months after the episode of acute haemolysis. A reticulocyte count should be performed before the G6PD assay to confirm that the child is not actively haemolysing RBCs.

Normocytic anaemia without reticulocytosis is due to transient erythroblastopenia of childhood (TEC), anaemia of chronic disease or rarely congenital dyserythropoietic anaemia (CDA) type 2. TEC should be suspected in an otherwise healthy child with normocytic anaemia and reticulocytopenia. In these children, extensive investigations are not necessary, provided that the blood film does not suggest RBC disorder or leukaemia.

When anaemia is associated with reductions in other cell lines, aplastic anaemia, hypersplenism or leukaemia should be suspected. In such instances, urgent bone marrow aspiration and biopsy are indicated.

Bone Marrow Aspiration and Biopsy

Bone marrow aspiration and biopsy are helpful to examine the erythropoiesis, granulopoiesis and thrombopoiesis as well as the entire bony trabecular architecture. Special tests, including cytogenetics, karyotyping and stains are used to arrive at a diagnosis, depending on the underlying condition. In aplastic anaemia, the bone marrow is hypocellular, and the marrow space is replaced by fat cells. Inherited marrow failure syndromes (e.g., Fanconi anaemia, Schwachmann Diamond syndrome) often show dysplastic features such as hyponucleated small megakaryocytes, multinucleated RBCs and hypolobulated and hypogranular myeloid cells. Leukaemia results in the replacement of the cellular component of the marrow by immature or undifferentiated cells.

INVESTIGATIONS OF MACROCYTIC ANAEMIA

The following investigations are helpful to arrive at a diagnosis in a child with macrocytic anaemia.

Blood Film

The presence of oval macrocytes and hyper segmented neutrophils suggests the possibility of megaloblastic anaemia due to folate or vitamin B12 deficiency.

Bone Marrow Aspiration and Biopsy

In megaloblastic anaemia, the bone marrow is hypercellular, with erythroid hyperplasia and giant metamyelocytes. Markedly reduced or virtually absent erythrocyte precursors in the marrow suggest pure red cell aplasia (e.g., Diamond Blackfan anaemia). Bone marrow erythroid hyperplasia, megaloblastosis and binucleated and multinucleated polychromatophilic erythroblasts are indicative of CDA.

Serum and Red Blood Cell Folate Levels

These will be low in the presence of folate deficiency.

Serum Vitamin B12 Levels

Serum vitamin B12 will be low in megaloblastic anaemia due to Vitamin B12 deficiency. RBC folate levels are also reduced in the presence of vitamin B12 deficiency.

Thyroid Function Test

This is important to exclude hypothyroidism as a cause for macrocytic anaemia.

Erythrocyte Adenosine Deaminase Activity

Erythrocyte adenosine deaminase activity is increased in most patients with Diamond Blackfan anaemia.

References

Lerner, Norma B. 2016. "The Anemias." In *Nelson Textbook of Pediatrics*, edited by Robert M. Kliegman, 2309-12. Philadelphia: Elsivier.

Mettananda, S., and D. G. de Silva. 2017. "Anaemia in children: are we using the correct prevention strategies?" *Ceylon Med J* 62 (2):73-76. doi: 10.4038/cmj.v62i2.8469.

Mettananda, S., and S. Wiliams. 2020. "Clinical and laboratory evaluation of childhood anaemia." *Sri Lanka Journal of Child Health* 49 (1):64-70.

Pippard, M. J. 2017. "Microcytic anaemias in childhood and iron-refractory iron deficiency anaemia." *Br J Haematol* 177 (2):167-168. doi: 10.1111/bjh.14558.

Weatherall, D. J., C. Hatton. 010. "Anaemia: pathophysiology, classification, and clinical features." In *Oxford Textbook of Medicine*, edited by D. A. Warrell, Cox, T. M., Firth, J. D. Oxford: Oxford University Press.

WHO. 2015. *The global prevalence of anaemia in 2011*. Geneva: World Health Organization.

PART 2.
MICROCYTIC ANAEMIAS

Chapter 3

IRON DEFICIENCY ANAEMIA

Sachith Mettananda*

Department of Paediatrics, University of Kelaniya, Ragama, Sri Lanka

Iron is an essential element for the cellular functions of the human body. It functions as an important co-factor of many enzymes due to its ability to mediate redox reactions through electron transfer between ferrous (Fe^{2+}) and ferric (Fe^{3+}) states. In addition to its primary role as a co-factor of haemoglobin, iron is a vital component in myoglobin and cytochrome enzymes.

IRON METABOLISM

The human body does not have a mechanism to excrete iron. Consequently, the iron balance is regulated at its absorption. This regulation is maintained by the hepatic protein hepcidin, which is the

* Corresponding Author's Email: sachith.mettananda@kln.ac.lk.

master regulator hormone of iron metabolism. The expression of hepcidin is increased in response to high circulating and tissue iron, inflammatory cytokines and metabolic needs. Hepcidin limits the iron entry into plasma by blocking and increasing degradation of its receptor ferroportin in the basolateral membrane of enterocytes and macrophages.

In iron deficiency, hepatic synthesis of hepcidin is suppressed by multiple factors that include decreased levels of iron-bound transferrin which leads to increased activity of the inhibitor transmembrane protease serine 6 (TMPRSS6) and erythroferrone which is secreted by erythroblasts in response to erythropoietin stimulation. The suppression of hepcidin enhances dietary iron absorption in the duodenum and release of iron from macrophages. In addition, hypoxia-inducible factor 2α increases the expression of duodenal divalent metal transporter 1 on the apical surface of enterocytes, thus increasing iron absorption (Figure 3.1).

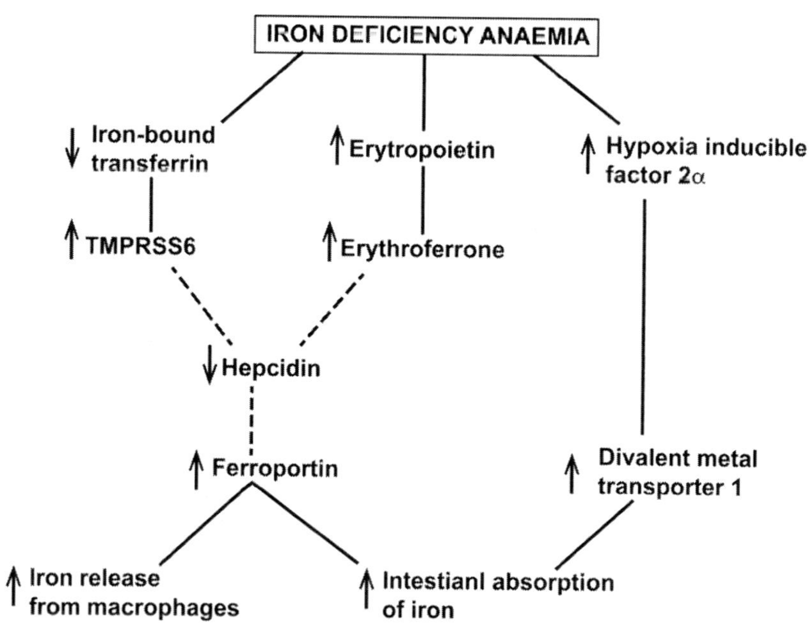

Figure 3.1. Iron regulation in iron deficiency anaemia. Intestinal iron absorption and iron mobilisation from macrophages are increased by the suppression of hepcidin. (Dashed lines indicate inhibitory pathways; TMPRSS6, Transmembrane protease serine 6).

Epidemiology

Iron deficiency is the most prevalent micronutrient deficiency in the world. It is estimated that iron deficiency accounts for approximately half of the patients with anaemia globally. The prevalence rates vary hugely in different regions of the world with a lower prevalence in Europe and North America and a higher prevalence in Africa and Asia. In children, the prevalence of iron deficiency is highest among preschool children who are aged between six months to five years.

Aetiology and Risk Factors

Iron deficiency in children has numerous causes. Dietary iron deficiency due to inadequate intake of iron-rich food is the most common cause in the developing world. In addition, decreased intestinal absorption due to coeliac disease or Crohn disease, increased gastrointestinal blood loss due to hookworm infections, cow's milk protein-induced colitis, Meckel's diverticulum, intestinal haemangioma or inflammatory bowel disease and increased iron requirement due to chronic infections are other less common causes. Also, rare inherited genetic mutations of proteins that are responsible for iron metabolism cause severe and refractory iron deficiency.

Iron deficiency is relatively uncommon in infants less than six months. Term infants have adequate iron stores at the time of birth due to maternal-to-fetal iron transfer during the third trimester. However, infants who are born prematurely or to mothers who are iron deficient are at risk of developing iron deficiency within the first six months of life. Similarly, the history of perinatal haemorrhage and being the donor of twin-to-twin transfusion syndrome are additional risk factors for iron deficiency in early infancy.

Stages and Classification

Iron deficiency has two distinct stages; iron deficiency and iron deficiency anaemia (IDA). Iron deficiency is the state of having inadequate body iron and iron stores to maintain normal physiological functions without associated low haemoglobin levels. When prolonged and untreated, iron deficiency leads to the state of IDA in which the child's haemoglobin level drops to sub-optimal levels for the age.

Clinical Manifestations

Clinical features of IDA could be divided into symptoms and signs that are due to iron deficiency itself or due to anaemia. Symptoms of iron deficiency include anorexia, fatigue, irritability, sleep disturbances, pica, pagophagia (desire to ingest ice) and behavioural changes. Physical signs of iron deficiency are angular stomatitis, glossitis, damaged hair and koilonychia. The clinical features of anaemia include dyspnoea, palpitations, headache, pallor, tachycardia and cardiac flow murmurs. When anaemia is very severe children develop cardiac failure.

Investigations and Diagnosis

Iron deficiency causes microcytic anaemia. Full blood count shows low haemoglobin (depending on the severity of anaemia) along with low MCV and MCH. The red cell distribution width is generally elevated. Blood film shows hypochromic and microcytic red blood cells (RBCs), pencil-shaped cells, teardrop cells and anisopoikilocytosis (Figure 2.4). Reactive thrombocytosis due to thrombopoietic activity of erythropoietin is common.

Diagnosis of iron deficiency is based on serum ferritin levels. Serum ferritin less than 15ng/dL is confirmatory of iron deficiency. As serum ferritin is an acute-phase reactant which can be elevated in the presence of infection, inflammation, liver diseases or malignancy, false-negative results with erroneously normal values are common. Some authorities recommend serum ferritin less than 30ng/dL as the cut-off value to diagnose mild iron deficiency. The other widely used test to confirm iron deficiency is transferrin saturation. The normal value for transferrin saturation is 30%, and iron deficiency is diagnosed when transferrin saturation drops below 16%. In addition, low serum ferritin, increased total iron-binding capacity, high soluble transferrin receptor level and high erythrocyte zinc protoporphyrin are suggestive of iron deficiency.

Another method of establishing the diagnosis of iron deficiency, especially in pre-school children in resource-poor countries, is to demonstrate a response to a therapeutic trial of iron. Here, children with anaemia are treated empirically with the treatment dose of iron and the response is assessed by repeating haemoglobin after one month. A rise of haemoglobin >1g/dL following 1-month treatment of iron confirms iron deficiency.

TREATMENT

The mainstay of treatment of IDA in children is oral iron therapy. Once the diagnosis is established, all children with IDA should be commenced on oral iron treatment with 3-6mg/kg/day of elemental iron. The amount of elemental iron available in different iron preparations vary. Therefore, it is essential that practising clinicians read the product information before prescribing iron treatment to children. Commonly used preparations contain ferrous sulphate (20-30% elemental iron per mg), ferrous fumarate (33% elemental iron per mg), ferrous gluconate (10-14% elemental iron per mg) and polysaccharide-iron complexes. Iron treatment can be given once daily or in 2-3 divided doses. For better absorption, iron should be taken at least 30 minutes before a meal. Absorption of iron is enhanced by vitamin C and is inhibited by calcium-containing meals; therefore, iron should be taken with fruit juice or water rather than milk.

Reported side effects of elemental iron are unpleasant taste, abdominal pain, constipation, diarrhoea and grey staining of teeth.

Dietary modifications to improve the consumption of iron-rich food is an essential part of the management. Meat, fish, poultry, liver, legumes, nuts and green vegetables are rich sources of iron. Food of animal origin contains haem iron which is easily absorbable and has high bioavailability (20-30%), whereas plant food contains non-haem iron with lower bioavailability (5-10%). Consumption of vitamin C containing food in the meal increases the absorption of non-haem iron. Tannins in tea and coffee and calcium in milk interferes with iron absorption, therefore, should not be consumed along with main meals.

Because the response to oral iron is rapid, intravenous iron is not routinely used in the management of iron deficiency in children. The rare indications for parenteral iron are intolerance or malabsorption of oral iron due to gastrointestinal diseases, for example, intestinal failure and inflammatory bowel disease. Similarly, blood transfusions are limited to children with impending cardiac failure due to severe IDA with very low haemoglobin (<5g/dL). Also, the routine prescription of vitamin C, folic acid or anthelminthic treatment is not indicated in the treatment of iron deficiency.

FOLLOW UP AND PROGNOSIS

Response to treatment of IDA is usually assessed by repeating the haemoglobin after one month. A rise in the haemoglobin of 1-2g/dL is indicative of an adequate response to iron. However, in situations where an early assessment is required, especially in severe IDA, an adequate response is indicated by a rise in reticulocyte count 3-7 days after starting iron treatment. In patients who have responded well, iron treatment should be continued for three months after haemoglobin and RBC indices have normalised. This is to ensure the replenishment of iron stores.

If the response to iron treatment is inadequate, several possibilities should be explored. After confirming that the dose and compliance are adequate, patients should be re-evaluated for non-dietary causes of iron deficiency, for example, malabsorption and chronic blood loss. Additionally, co-existing haemoglobinopathies (see chapter 4) and genetic diseases causing iron refractory iron deficiency anaemia (see chapter 6) should be considered.

PREVENTION

Prevention of iron deficiency and IDA has been a topic for debate for many years. Non-anaemic iron deficiency has shown to adversely affect the neurodevelopmental outcome of children in psychomotor and mental development, social-emotional behaviour, attention span and mathematical skills. It has also been linked to increased incidence of attention deficit hyperactivity disorder and autistic spectrum disorder. Due to this, some advocate universal supplementation with elemental iron 1-3mg/kg/day for children. However, there is no consensus on this. Taking a diet rich in iron to fulfil the recommended dietary allowance (1mg/kg/day in infancy and 7-10mg/day during childhood) is universally accepted.

RECENT ADVANCES

Regulation of iron metabolism and iron deficiency are rapidly advancing fields. Recent advances are made both in the diagnosis and management of IDA. It is known that serum hepcidin levels are low in IDA. Recent research shows that the assay of serum hepcidin will provide accurate information on the iron status of the body. Additionally, identification and development of biomarkers to detect tissue-specific iron deficiency, especially in the skeletal muscle and heart are ongoing.

Regarding the treatment of iron deficiency, increasing evidence shows that low dose (elemental iron 3mg/kg/day) iron treatment is effective and better tolerated than higher doses (elemental iron 6mg/kg/day). Because absorption of non-haem iron is low (5%-28%) higher doses result in the generation of reactive oxygen species by non-absorbed iron on the intestinal mucosa. Also, there is increasing evidence to suggest that non-absorbed iron alters the composition of the gut microbiome with reduction of beneficial *Lactobacillus* and *Bifidobacterium* bacteria, thus enhancing the growth of pathogens. There is ongoing work on the development of iron salts which are better tolerated; sucrosomial iron, haem iron polypeptide and iron-containing nanoparticles are few examples.

REFERENCES

Allen, A., S. Perera, L. Perera, R. Rodrigo, S. Mettananda, A. Matope, I. Silva, N. Hameed, C. A. Fisher, N. Olivieri, D. J. Weatherall, S. Allen, and A. Premawardhena. 2019. "A "One-Stop" Screening Protocol for Haemoglobinopathy Traits and Iron Deficiency in Sri Lanka." *Front Mol Biosci* 6:66. doi: 10.3389/fmolb.2019.00066.

Camaschella, C. 2015. "Iron-deficiency anemia." *N Engl J Med* 372 (19):1832-43. doi: 10.1056/NEJMra1401038.

Camaschella, C. 2017. "New insights into iron deficiency and iron deficiency anemia." *Blood Rev* 31 (4):225-233. doi: 10.1016/j.blre. 2017.02.004.

Camaschella, C. 2019. "Iron deficiency." *Blood* 133 (1):30-39. doi: 10. 1182/blood-2018-05-815944.

Cappellini, M. D., K. M. Musallam, and A. T. Taher. 2020. "Iron deficiency anaemia revisited." *J Intern Med* 287 (2):153-170. doi: 10. 1111/joim.13004.

Jonker, F. A. M., E. Te Poel, I. Bates, and M. Boele van Hensbroek. 2017. "Anaemia, iron deficiency and susceptibility to infection in children in sub-Saharan Africa, guideline dilemmas." *Br J Haematol* 177 (6):878-883. doi: 10.1111/bjh.14593.

Lopez, A., P. Cacoub, I. C. Macdougall, and L. Peyrin-Biroulet. 2016. "Iron deficiency anaemia." *Lancet* 387 (10021):907-16. doi: 10.1016/ S0140-6736(15)60865-0.

Mattiello, V., M. Schmugge, H. Hengartner, N. von der Weid, and R. Renella. 2020. "Diagnosis and management of iron deficiency in children with or without anemia: consensus recommendations of the SPOG Pediatric Hematology Working Group." *Eur J Pediatr* 179 (4):527-545. doi: 10.1007/s00431-020-03597-5.

Mettananda, S., and D. G. de Silva. 2017. "Anaemia in children: are we using the correct prevention strategies?" *Ceylon Med J* 62 (2):73-76. doi: 10.4038/cmj.v62i2.8469.

Mettananda, S., S. Paranamana, R. Fernando, M. Suranjan, R. Rodrigo, L. Perera, T. Vipulaguna, P. Fernando, M. Fernando, Bktp Dayanath, Y. Costa, and A. Premawardhena. 2020. "Microcytic anemia in children: parallel screening for iron deficiency and thalassemia provides a useful opportunity for thalassemia prevention in low- and middle-income countries." *Pediatr Hematol Oncol*:1-11. doi: 10.1080/08880018.2020. 1725200.

Mettananda, S., M. Suranjan, R. Fernando, T. Dias, C. Mettananda, R. Rodrigo, L. Perera, R. Gibbons, A. Premawardhena, and D. Higgs. 2018. "Anaemia among females in child-bearing age: Relative contributions, effects and interactions of alpha- and beta-thalassaemia." *PLoS One* 13 (11):e0206928. doi: 10.1371/journal. pone.0206928.

Pivina, L., Y. Semenova, M. D. Doşa, M. Dauletyarova, and G. Bjørklund. 2019. "Iron Deficiency, Cognitive Functions, and Neurobehavioral Disorders in Children." *J Mol Neurosci* 68 (1):1-10. doi: 10.1007/ s12031-019-01276-1.

Chapter 4

THALASSAEMIA

Sachith Mettananda[*]

Department of Paediatrics, University of Kelaniya, Ragama, Sri Lanka

Thalassaemia was first described by the American paediatrician Thomas Cooley in 1925. The term 'thalassaemia' was derived from the Greek word '*thalassa*' which means 'sea' and 'anaemia' because the disease was initially reported in regions adjacent to the Mediterranean Sea. Alternatively, thalassaemia is known as Cooley's anaemia.

EPIDEMIOLOGY

Thalassaemia is one of the most prevalent genetic diseases in the world, with an annual incidence of 70,000 births globally. The highest prevalence is reported in the tropical 'thalassemia belt' which extends from the Mediterranean region through sub-Saharan Africa and the Middle East

[*] Corresponding Author's Email: sachith.mettananda@kln.ac.lk.

to South and South-East Asia. However, due to recent migration, thalassaemia is frequently reported in Northern Europe and North America as well.

Genetic Basis

Adult haemoglobin, HbA is a tetramer of two α-globin and two β-globin polypeptide chains each combined with a haem moiety. Autosomal recessive genetic mutations that result in reduced synthesis of these globin chains cause thalassaemia. Mutations of the α-globin gene results in decreased synthesis of α-globin chains and α-thalassaemia, whereas mutations in the β-globin gene leads to reduced synthesis of β-globin chains and β-thalassaemia.

α-Thalassaemia is caused by over 120 mutations of α-globin genes which are located in chromosome 16. Most of these mutations are deletions involving variable lengths of the α-globin gene locus (Table 4.1). Normal individuals have four copies of the α-globin gene, two on each chromosome (denoted as 'αα/αα'), and deletion can either remove one or both genes from a chromosome. Deletions which involve both α-globin genes (denoted as '--') and completely abolish the expression from a single chromosome are known as α^0-thalassaemia, whereas deletions which remove one gene (denoted as '-α' or 'α-') and partially downregulate expression from a chromosome are known as α^+-thalassaemia. Rarely, deletions of the upstream enhancer elements that are essential for the expression of α-globin genes cause α-thalassaemia despite having normal genes. Additionally, a small proportion of patients with α-thalassaemia has non-deletional point mutations of the α-globin gene.

Over 300 mutations of the β-globin gene located in chromosome 11 are known to cause β-thalassaemia. Most of these are point mutations either in the gene or flanking regions. β-Thalassaemia mutations are categorized into β^0-, β^+- and β^{++}-thalassaemia alleles depending on the extent to which the β-globin chain output is reduced. Mutations that completely abolish the production of β-globin are known as β^0-thalassaemia (severe) whilst mutations which result in a milder reduction in β-globin are known as β^+-thalassaemia. A group of mutations which are labelled as β^{++}-thalassaemia results in only subtle effects on the production of β-globin chains. In addition, a point mutation at codon 26 of the β-globin gene results in structurally abnormal β-globin protein (β^E) which is synthesised at reduced rates to give rise to the phenotype of β-thalassemia. The haemoglobin molecule which is composed of α- and β^E-globin chains is labelled as haemoglobin E (HbE, $\alpha_2\beta^E{}_2$).

PATHOPHYSIOLOGY

The synthesis of α- and β-globin chains in normal healthy red blood cells (RBCs) occur in a coordinated manner to maintain a precise balance between two types of globin chains to prevent excess accumulation of one over the other. In thalassaemia, the synthesis of either α- or β-globin is reduced or completely abolished resulting in accumulation of other types of globin chains in RBCs. α-Thalassaemia leads to the excess synthesis of β- and γ-globin chains whilst β-thalassaemia results in accumulation of α-globin chains. Molecular pathology of thalassaemia is triggered by these excess globin chains. In β-thalassaemia, excess free α-globin chains precipitate in RBCs and their precursors leading to the formation of toxic α-hemichromes and reactive oxygen species resulting in oxidative destruction of erythroid cells. Destruction of mature RBCs in the circulation leads to haemolysis and erythroid precursors within bone marrow lead to ineffective erythropoiesis. The clinically significant anaemia in thalassaemia is a cumulative effect of ineffective erythropoiesis, premature haemolysis and direct reduction of haemoglobin synthesis.

CLASSIFICATION

Clinical phenotype of thalassaemia can be classified based on its genotype. α-Thalassaemia is classified depending on the number α-globin genes mutated (Table 4.1). Mutation of one or two α-globin genes is known as α-thalassaemia trait whereas mutations of three α-globin genes lead to the formation of haemoglobin H (HbH, β-globin tetramers) in RBCs, therefore, is referred to as HbH disease. Mutation of all four α-globin genes leads to complete absence of α-globin synthesis and accumulation of γ-globin tetramers (haemoglobin Bart's) in erythroid cells from fetal life thus is known as haemoglobin Bart's hydrops fetalis syndrome.

Table 4.1. Genotype-phenotype correlation of thalassaemia

	Genotype/s	Phenotype
α-thalassaemia		
One α-globin gene mutation	- α/αα	α-Thalassaemia trait
Two α-globin gene mutation	- α/- α, - -/αα,	α-Thalassaemia trait
Three α-globin gene mutation	- -/- α	Haemoglobin H disease
Four α-globin gene mutation	- -/- -	Haemoglobin Bart's hydrops fetalis
β-thalassaemia		
Heterozygous β-thalassaemia mutation	β/β^0, β/β^+, β/β^{++}	β-Thalassaemia trait
Homozygous/ compound heterozygous β-thalassaemia mutation	β^0/β^0, β^+/β^+, β^0/β^+	β-Thalassaemia major
Compound heterozygous for β-thalassaemia and haemoglobin E mutation	β^E/β^0, β^E/β^+, β^E/β^{++}	Haemoglobin E β-thalassaemia

Similarly, β-thalassaemia can be classified as β-thalassaemia trait, β-thalassaemia major and β-thalassaemia intermedia. Heterozygous mutation of the β-globin gene causes β-thalassaemia trait whilst homozygous (same mutation in both alleles) and compound heterozygous (different mutations in two alleles) mutations result in β-thalassaemia major. β-Thalassaemia intermedia is a phenotype with intermediate severity due to coinheritance of genetic modifiers that ameliorates the severity (e.g., α-thalassaemia or hereditary persistence of fetal haemoglobin) in a child who otherwise have a β-thalassaemia major phenotype (Table 4.2). Alternatively, it can be produced in a child with heterozygous β-thalassaemia mutation with excess α-globin genes. Co-inheritance of a β-thalassaemia allele from one parent and β^E allele from the other parents results in HbE β-thalassaemia.

Table 4.2. Genetic modifiers of β-thalassaemia

	Factors that ameliorate the severity of homozygous or compound heterozygous β-thalassaemia	Factors that worsen the severity of heterozygous β-thalassaemia
β-Thalassaemia mutation	Milder (β^+ or β^{++}) mutations	Dominantly inherited β-thalassaemia mutations
α-globin genotype	Coinheritance of α-thalassaemia (- α/αα, -α/- α or - -/αα)	Coinheritance of excess α-globin genes (ααα/αα, ααα/ααα or αααα/αα)
Increased synthesis of γ-globin and haemoglobin F	$\delta\beta^0$-thalassaemia *Xmn1-HBG2* Polymorphisms *BCL11A* Polymorphisms Polymorphisms at *HBS1L-MYB* intergenic region or *MYB* *KLF1* mutations	

Thalassaemia is also classified based on the clinical severity into three groups. The mildest group is thalassaemia trait which is composed of asymptomatic individuals with α- or β-thalassaemia trait. The most severely affected children who require regular blood transfusions are classified as transfusion-dependent thalassaemia. This group consists of patients with β-thalassaemia major, severe HbE β-thalassaemia and survivors of haemoglobin Bart's hydrops fetalis syndrome. All other patients who require infrequent or occasional transfusions are classified as non-transfusion dependent thalassaemia. β-Thalassaemia intermedia, mild to moderate HbE β-thalassaemia and HbH disease comprise this group.

CLINICAL MANIFESTATIONS

Children with β-thalassaemia are asymptomatic at birth. This is because, at the time of birth, the predominant type of haemoglobin is haemoglobin F (HbF) and the synthesis of HbA occurs only at low levels. Physiological switch of haemoglobin from HbF to HbA happens around the age of six months at which the patients with transfusion-dependent β-thalassaemia become progressively anaemic and manifest clinical features. Symptoms of β-thalassaemia include lethargy, poor feeding, irritability, fatigability, growth faltering and shortness of breath. The characteristic physical signs are pallor, mild jaundice, signs of extramedullary haematopoiesis which include hepatomegaly and splenomegaly and signs of bone marrow expansion, for example, frontal bossing, maxillary hyperplasia and dental malocclusion.

In contrast, patients with haemoglobin Bart's hydrops fetalis manifest clinical features in utero. They develop severe intrauterine anaemia due to the absence of α-globin, which is required to form HbF. The clinical features are massive hepatosplenomegaly, cardiac failure, gross generalized body oedema, enlargement of the placenta and eventual intrauterine death. Due to advances in fetal medicine and intrauterine transfusions, some babies survive. These survivors have transfusion-dependent thalassaemia and congenital malformation due to fetal hypoxia including congenital heart diseases, urogenital abnormalities, limb deformities and intellectual retardation.

Patients with non-transfusion dependent thalassaemia have a less severe phenotype and manifest milder clinical features of anaemia usually after two years of age. The physical signs are similar to transfusion-dependent thalassaemia and include pallor, mild jaundice, hepatomegaly, splenomegaly and features of bone marrow expansion.

INVESTIGATIONS AND DIAGNOSIS

Once β-thalassaemia is clinically suspected, the initial evaluation includes a full blood count and a peripheral blood film. The full blood count shows low haemoglobin, low MCV and low MCH. MCHC is low or low-normal. Blood film shows microcytosis, hypochromia, anisopoikilocytosis and nucleated RBCs (Figure 2.4). The diagnosis of β-thalassaemia is confirmed by qualitative and quantitative haemoglobin analysis by high-performance liquid chromatography (HPLC) or capillary electrophoresis (Table 4.3).

Table 4.3. Quantification of haemoglobin subtypes in β-thalassaemia

	HbA	HbA_2	HbF	HbE
Normal	>95%	<3.4%	<2%	-
β-Thalassaemia trait	>90%	3.5-7.0%	1-3%	-
β^0/β^0-Thalassaemia major	-	2–5%	95–98%	-
β^0/β^+-Thalassaemia major or β^+/β^+-thalassaemia major	10–30%	2–5%	70–90%	-
HbE β-thalassaemia	<10%	<3.4%	30-70%	30-50%

Full blood count report of a patient with α-thalassaemia is indistinguishable from that of β-thalassaemia with low haemoglobin, MCV and MCH. Findings in blood film are also similar. Patients with HbH disease show HbH inclusion bodies in the supravital staining of peripheral blood film with characteristic golf-ball like appearance of cells due to regularly distributed stippling over blue-stained background when stained with 1% Brilliant Cresyl Blue (Figure 2.4). The confirmatory diagnosis of α-thalassaemia can only be made by DNA analysis using multiplex gap-PCR, multiplex ligation-dependent probe amplification, direct sequencing of PCR amplified α-gene fragments or next-generation sequencing.

TREATMENT

The mainstay of treatment of thalassaemia is blood transfusion to correct anaemia, suppress bone marrow and extramedullary erythropoietic activity, promote optimal growth and allow normal physical activity. The transfusion protocol and frequency depend on whether the patient has transfusion-dependent or non-transfusion dependent thalassaemia, which should be decided during the first few years of treatment. However, this categorisation will require frequent revisiting throughout life as patients can shift from transfusion-dependent to non-transfusion dependent category and *vice versa*. Patients with transfusion-dependent thalassaemia should be transfused 2-5 weekly with leuco-depleted packed RBCs which are less than two weeks old to maintain a pre-transfusion haemoglobin level of 9.0–10.5g/dL. In contrast, patients with non-transfusion dependent thalassaemia do not require regular transfusions. Lower baseline haemoglobin levels (as low as 6-7g/dL) are acceptable in these patients; indications for transfusion are growth failure, reduced exercise tolerance, poor quality of life and rapidly enlarging spleen (>3cm per year).

Due to regular transfusions and increased intestinal iron absorption related to inappropriate suppression of hepatic synthesis of hepcidin, iron overload is an inevitable complication of thalassaemia. Screening for iron overload by monitoring serum ferritin commences when patients receive 6-8 transfusions and should be continued 3-monthly. In addition, several MRI based techniques are available to determine organ-specific iron overload. Nonetheless, serum ferritin >1000ng/mL is considered as the indication to commence iron chelation using monotherapy or combination of iron chelator medication; desferrioxamine, deferiprone or deferasirox. Desferrioxamine is the most effective iron chelator, however, requires intravenous or subcutaneous infusion for long hours. Deferasirox is an oral chelator with equal efficacy to desferrioxamine, which has now become the first line iron chelator in many countries worldwide. Deferiprone is less efficacious, however, has an ability to selectively chelate myocardial iron.

Though splenectomy was routinely performed as an adjunct to transfusion therapy in the past, it is rarely performed at present due to high incidence of post-splenectomy adverse events that include sepsis, leg ulcers, pulmonary hypertension, venous thrombosis and strokes. Current indications for splenectomy are limited to hypersplenism, symptomatic splenomegaly and requirement of very high transfusion volumes (>200-250 mL/kg/year).

The only curative treatment available for thalassaemia at present is allogenic haematopoietic stem cell (HSC) transplantation. The best outcome is reported when transplanting HSCs from HLA-matched sibling donors, which has an overall survival of 90% and disease-free survival of 80%. Other less optimal options available for patients who do not have matched sibling donors are to use HSCs from matched-unrelated donors, haploidentical related donors, HLA-mismatched family members or umbilical cord blood. Serious adverse events of HSC transplantation that include transplant-related mortality, graft-versus-host disease and graft failure are important limitations of the procedure.

COMPLICATIONS

β-Thalassaemia is a chronic progressive disease with multiple long-term complications related to chronic anaemia, blood transfusions, iron overload and iron chelator medications. Therefore, continuous surveillance of complications is pivotal to provide optimal care for patients with thalassaemia (Table 4.4).

FOLLOW UP AND PROGNOSIS

Patients with transfusion-dependent thalassaemia who are managed only with supportive therapy have a life expectancy up to 40-60 years depending on the availability of safe blood products and other health facilities. However, poor quality of life and psychological morbidities are commonly reported among them. The commonest cause of death is cardiac failure due to iron overload.

Table 4.4. Monitoring and treatment of complications of thalassaemia

Complication	Methods of evaluation	Treatment
Cardiac dysfunction	Cardiac MRI, echocardiography	ACE inhibitors, diuretics, intensive iron chelation
Hepatic fibrosis and cirrhosis	Hepatic transaminases, abdominal ultrasonography, liver MRI	Standard management of chronic liver disease
Short stature	Height velocity	Growth hormone (only if deficient)
Delayed puberty	Tanner staging, gonadotrophins, testosterone or oestrogen	Hormone replacement therapy
Hypothyroidism	Thyroid function tests	Levothyroxine
Hypoparathyroidism	Serum calcium, phosphate, parathyroid hormone level	25-hydroxyvitamin D, calcium supplements and phosphate binders
Diabetes mellitus	Fasting blood glucose, fructosamine	Oral hypoglycaemic drugs, insulin
Osteoporosis	Bone densitometry, dual-energy x-ray absorptiometry scan	Vitamin D, calcium, bisphosphonates
Viral hepatitis	Hepatitis B surface antigen, hepatitis C RNA, anti-hepatitis C antibody	Hepatitis B - interferon and antivirals Hepatitis C - direct-acting antivirals
Pulmonary hypertension	Tricuspid regurgitant jet velocity	Sildenafil, bosentan
Cerebrovascular events	MRA brain	Antiplatelet prophylaxis
Venous thrombosis		Anticoagulant therapy

FAMILY SCREENING AND GENETIC COUNSELLING

Parents of children with severe forms of thalassaemia, both β-thalassaemia major and haemoglobin Bart's hydrops fetalis, should be screened for identification of thalassaemia trait and carrier status. Once confirmed, the couples in which both partners are carrying β-thalassaemia mutations should be counselled regarding the recurrence risk of 25% in future pregnancies. In families where both partners are carriers for α^0-thalassaemia mutation, genetic counselling should be performed regarding the 25% risk of a pregnancy with haemoglobin Bart's hydrops fetalis which carry a high risk for both the fetus and the mother. If facilities and legal provisions are available, these couples should be offered antenatal diagnosis and termination in the case of an affected offspring.

PREVENTION

Main aspects of a thalassaemia prevention program are to identify thalassaemia carriers by community screening to prevent at-risk marriages between two carriers, identification of at-risk couples and provide counselling regarding the risk of affected conceptions and provision of antenatal diagnosis and termination if legal provisions are available. Identification of thalassaemia carriers in a community is made by detecting microcytosis in full blood counts followed by haemoglobin HPLC or capillary electrophoresis for β-thalassaemia carriers and DNA analysis for α-thalassaemia carriers.

RECENT ADVANCES

Several novel pharmacological and genetic-based therapies are being investigated as treatment options for β-thalassaemia at present. Most of these treatment strategies aim to restore α/β-like globin chain imbalance in β-thalassaemia RBCs. Induction of γ-globin and HbF by hydroxyurea and improving ineffective erythropoiesis by inhibiting its mediators using luspatercept (activin type IIB receptor-ligand trap) and ruxolitinib (JAK2 inhibitor) are being evaluated in clinical trials.

Gene therapy which uses harvesting of HSCs from patients with β-thalassaemia, insertion of the normal β-globin gene using viral vectors *in vitro* and transplanting the HSCs with normal β-globin gene back to the patient as an autologous HSC transplantation has successfully cured several patients with β-thalassaemia in clinical trials. Additionally, extremely novel genome editing approaches to improve the globin balance either by upregulating γ-globin or downregulating α-globin are approaching clinical trials.

References

Cappellini, M. D., J. B. Porter, V. Viprakasit, and A. T. Taher. 2018. "A paradigm shift on beta-thalassaemia treatment: How will we manage this old disease with new therapies?" *Blood Rev* 32 (4):300-311. doi: 10.1016/j.blre.2018.02.001.

Cappellini, M. D., A. Cohen, J. Porter, A. Taher, and V. Viprakasit. 2014. *Guidelines for the management of transfusion dependent thalassaemia (TDT)* Edited by M. D. Cappellini, A. Cohen, J. Porter, A. Taher and V. Viprakasit. 3rd Edition ed. Cyprus: Thalassaemia International Federation.

Higgs, D. R. 2013. "The molecular basis of alpha-thalassemia." *Cold Spring Harb Perspect Med* 3 (1):a011718. doi: 10.1101/cshperspect.a011718.

Mettananda, S., R. J. Gibbons, and D. R. Higgs. 2016. "Understanding alpha-globin gene regulation and implications for the treatment of beta-thalassemia." *Ann N Y Acad Sci* 1368 (1):16-24. doi: 10.1111/nyas.12988.

Mettananda, S., and D. R. Higgs. 2018. "Molecular Basis and Genetic Modifiers of Thalassemia." *Hematol Oncol Clin North Am* 32 (2):177-191. doi: 10.1016/j.hoc.2017.11.003.

Piel, F. B., and D. J. Weatherall. 2014. "The alpha-Thalassemias." *New England Journal of Medicine* 371 (20):1908-1916. doi: doi 10.1056/Nejmra1404415.

Taher, A. T., D. J. Weatherall, and M. D. Cappellini. 2018. "Thalassaemia." *Lancet* 391 (10116):155-167. doi: 10.1016/S0140-6736(17)31822-6.

Taher, A., E. Vichinsky, K. Musallam, M. D. Cappellini, and V. Viprakasit. 2013. *Guidelines for the management of non transfusion dependent thalassaemia (NTDT)* Cyprus: Thalassaemia International Federation.

Weatherall, D. J., and J. B. Clegg. 2001. *The thalassaemia syndromes*. 4 ed. Oxford: Blackwell Science.

Chapter 5

SICKLE CELL DISEASE

Sachith Mettananda*

Department of Paediatrics, University of Kelaniya, Ragama, Sri Lanka

Sickle cell disease (SCD) is the most common genetic disease in the world. It comprises a number of clinical conditions with variable severity ranging from asymptomatic to severe debilitating disease. The hallmark of SCD is the presence of abnormal sickle haemoglobin, HbS, in red blood cells (RBCs).

EPIDEMIOLOGY

The annual incidence of SCD is estimated to be 300,000 worldwide. It is highly prevalent in tropical regions of sub-Saharan Africa, Mediterranean, middle east and south Asia. This is due to the protective advantage of heterozygous carrier state of SCD against *Plasmodium*

* Corresponding Author's Email: sachith.mettananda@kln.ac.lk.

falciparum malaria, which has been a highly prevalent fatal disease in this part of the world. However, due to recent migration, SCD has become common in Europe and North America as well.

Genetic Basis

SCD is caused by an autosomal recessively inherited point mutation in the β-globin gene located on chromosome 11. This mutation involves a substitution of adenine to thymine in the β-globin gene (β^S allele). The resultant change in the codon replaces amino acid glutamic acid with valine at position six of the β-globin chain generating an abnormal β-globin (*HBB* Glu6Val). The association of these mutant β-globin chains with α-globin chains forms tetramers of abnormal haemoglobin, HbS.

The inheritance of β^S allele in the heterozygous state is clinically asymptomatic and is termed sickle cell trait or sickle cell carrier. SCD refers to any clinical condition in which the β^S allele is co-inherited with a mutation of the other β-globin allele that reduces normal β-globin production. The presence of β^S in both alleles of β-globin gene results in homozygous SCD, which is known as sickle cell anaemia (SCA). Additionally, β^S allele can be co-inherited with a number of mutations in the other β-globin allele. These compound heterozygous states that cause haemoglobin SC disease (heterozygosity for HbS and HbC), haemoglobin SE disease (heterozygosity for HbS and HbE) and sickle β-thalassaemia (heterozygosity for HbS and β-thalassaemia) results in SCD of intermediate severity.

Pathophysiology

The pathophysiology of SCD is complex. During deoxygenated state, HbS polymerizes intracellularly causing erythrocytes to undergo a rapid but reversible change in shape from normal flexible biconcave contour to an elongated rigid form. These abnormal (sickled) erythrocytes cause organ damage by two main mechanisms (Figure 5.1). Firstly, polymerisation of HbS causes oxidative damage to the erythrocyte membrane leading to both intravascular and extravascular haemolysis. This leads to anaemia and related complications of SCD. Secondly, sickled erythrocytes block small blood vessels causing vaso-occlusion leading to a range of acute and chronic complications of repeated ischaemia. Several cellular and plasma factors and abnormal endothelial interactions contribute to vaso-occlusion. Intravascular haemolysis releases free haem and haemoglobin and other vasoactive substances which lead to depletion of nitric oxide resulting in vasoconstriction and activation of platelets and coagulation factors to contribute to vaso-occlusion. In addition, activation of endothelial cells, triggering of the inflammatory cascade and increased neutrophil adhesiveness worsen vaso-occlusion.

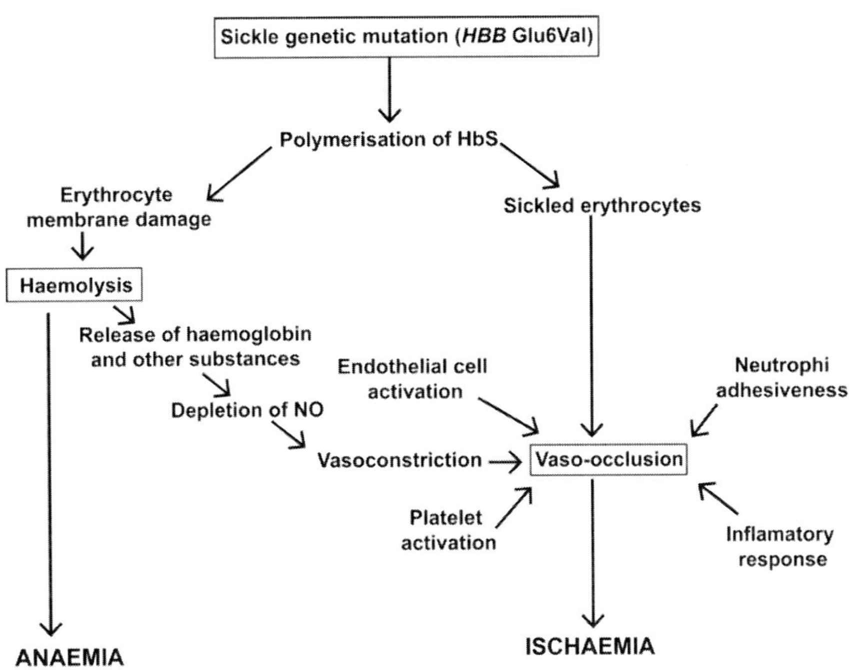

Figure 5.1. Pathophysiology of sickle cell disease. The polymerisation of HbS leads to sickling and membrane damage of erythrocytes to cause haemolysis and vaso-occlusion.

GENETIC MODIFIERS

Being a prototype autosomal recessive genetic disease, one would expect SCD to follow the normal Mendelian inheritance pattern with distinct clinical phenotypes. However, it is not the case. A number of other genetic and environmental modifiers alter the disease phenotype even in patients with identical genetic mutations. Fetal haemoglobin (HbF) interrupts the polymerization of HbS therefore, increasing the HbF content in RBCs decreases the severity of SCD. HbS mutation is inherited along with different haplotypes of the β-globin gene cluster, which is associated with variable levels of expression of γ-globin and thus HbF. Arab-Indian and Senegal haplotypes are associated with high levels of HbF (10-15%), and milder phenotype, whereas Benin and Bantu haplotypes are associated with low HbF (6-8%) and severe phenotypes. Similarly, genetic polymorphisms of the *BCL11A* and *MYB* genes are associated with high HbF and milder clinical phenotype of SCD. Also, co-inheritance of α-thalassaemia trait (deletion of one or two out of four α-globin genes) reduces the amount of HbS which mitigate the erythrocyte damage, thus resulting in less severe phenotype.

CLINICAL MANIFESTATIONS

SCD affects every system of the body. Its clinical manifestations result from ischemia due to vaso-occlusion, haemolytic anaemia or both. Acute complications of SCD are usually caused by vaso-occlusion of which acute vaso-occlusive pain is the commonest. It is characterized by severe unremitting pain in any part of the body but most often in the chest, abdomen or extremities. Although this can be triggered by infection, dehydration, stress, cold, wind and low humidity, precipitants are not identified in many.

Acute chest syndrome is possibly the most fatal complication of SCD. It is characterised by fever, cough, wheezing, chest pain, respiratory distress and hypoxemia associated with infiltrates in chest radiographs. The aetiology of acute chest syndrome is multifactorial, which includes infection, vaso-occlusion and thromboembolism.

Infection is another common cause of morbidity and mortality in SCD. Patients with SCD are at risk of developing infections, specifically by encapsulated bacteria (*Streptococcus pneumoniae*, *Haemophilus influenzae* type b and *Neisseria meningitidis*) due to splenic dysfunction and functional asplenia following repeated splenic infarcts. Common infections are septicaemia, meningitis, pneumonia, osteomyelitis and septic arthritis.

Nervous system manifestations of SCD could be acute or chronic. These patients are at risk of developing ischemic as well as haemorrhagic strokes which present as acute onset weakness, hemiplegia or cranial nerve palsies. Other nervous system manifestations of the disease include transient ischemic attacks, silent cerebral infarctions, seizures, headaches, cerebral venous thrombosis and posterior reversible encephalopathy syndrome.

SCD is characterised by chronic compensated anaemia which can sometimes have acute worsening. Acute worsening could occur due to several reasons. An aplastic crisis is characterised by a sudden transient arrest of erythropoiesis typically caused by infection (most commonly parvovirus B19) which lead to severe anaemia that lasts for 2-14 days. Splenic sequestration with pooling of large volumes of blood with rapidly enlarging spleen can occur in younger children giving rise to acute anaemia and hypovolaemic shock. Although rare, hyperhaemolysis is another cause for acute anaemia in children with SCD. Excessive haemolysis of transfused cells, as well as the patient's own RBCs following delayed haemolytic transfusion reaction, is the cause for hyperhaemolysis.

Other acute manifestations of SCD are dactylitis, avascular necrosis, renal infarctions, myocardial infarction and priapism. Chronic complications of the disease include leg ulcers, restrictive lung disease, pulmonary hypertension, hyposthenuria (renal concentration defects), chronic kidney disease, diastolic dysfunction, pigment gall stones and retinopathy.

INVESTIGATIONS AND DIAGNOSIS

Clinical features of SCD are not present at birth. This is because the expression of β-globin gene is relatively low at the time of birth. Depending on the prevalence and health policy of a country, SCD is either diagnosed at routine neonatal screening or during early childhood after manifestation of clinical features.

Universal newborn screening for SCD is practised in some countries like UK and USA whereas selected screening of at-risk pregnancies is done in countries like India. Either way, newborn babies are screened soon after birth by haemoglobin subtype protein analysis methods such as haemoglobin electrophoresis, isoelectric focusing or high-performance liquid chromatography (HPLC). The presence of FS pattern with predominantly HbF, a small amount of HbS and the absence of HbA confirms homozygous SCA.

In countries where neonatal screening is not available, the diagnosis of SCD is generally made during the second year of life when children present with clinical manifestations. Preliminary investigations of these patients will reveal mild to moderate anaemia, reticulocytosis (3-15%), unconjugated hyperbilirubinemia, elevated lactate dehydrogenase and low serum haptoglobin. Blood film will show sickled RBCs, polychromasia and Howell-Jolly bodies. Confirmation of the diagnosis is by haemoglobin subtype quantification methods; either capillary electrophoresis or HPLC (Table 5.1).

Table 5.1. Quantification of haemoglobin subtypes in sickle cell disease

	HbA	HbS	HbC	HbF	HbA_2
Normal	>95%	0	0	<2%	<3.4%
Sickle trait	50-70%	20-40%	0	1-3%	<3.4%
Haemoglobin C trait	50-70%	0	20-40%	1-3%	<3.4%
Sickle cell anaemia	0	80-95%	0	5%-15%	<3.4%
Haemoglobin SC disease	0	50-55%	40-45%	1-3%	<3.4%
Sickle β-thalassaemia	<30%	50-80%	0	<20%	<7.0%

TREATMENT

Treatment of SCD requires individualised care by a multidisciplinary team. Components of management include general treatment modalities, treatment of organ-specific manifestations, prevention of complications and potentially curative therapies.

Oral hydroxyurea (also known as hydroxycarbamide) is the mainstay of treatment of SCD at present. It is recommended to all children with SCD; however, the extent of its use depends on the region and the country. Hydroxyurea has shown to increase HbF and reduce the incidence of vaso-occlusive events, hospitalizations and mortality of patients with SCD. Important side effects of hydroxyurea include neutropenia, thrombocytepenia, gastrointestinal disturbances and elevation of hepatic transaminases.

Most patients with SCD do not require regular blood transfusions. However, blood transfusions help to improve haemoglobin, decrease the percentage of HbS, suppress the formation of sickled erythrocytes, increase haemoglobin oxygen saturation and reduce the risk of vaso-occlusion. Indications for acute therapeutic transfusions are symptomatic anaemia, acute stroke, acute chest syndrome, multiorgan failure, acute aplastic crisis and splenic sequestration. Acute transfusions are either given as simple blood transfusions or exchange transfusions (by removing some of the patient's blood) to increase the haemoglobin to above 10g/dL while maintaining HbS below 30%. Prophylactic transfusions are indicated pre-operatively to patients who are undergoing surgery. Chronic regular preventive transfusions are indicated in secondary prevention of stroke, acute chest syndrome, recurrent priapism and pulmonary hypertension. The goals of chronic regular transfusions are to maintain HbS below 30% and haemoglobin above 9g/dL.

Prevention of infection is another important aspect in the management of SCD. All patients should receive immunisation against *Streptococcus pneumoniae*, *Neisseria meningitidis, Haemophilus influenzae* type b and seasonal influenza in addition to routine vaccines. Prophylactic twice-daily oral penicillin is indicated in all children with SCD at least until five years of age. Treatment of other organ-specific complications is summarised in Table 5.2.

Table 5.2. Treatment of common organ-specific manifestations of sickle cell disease

Organ system	Manifestation	Treatment
Pain	Vaso-occlusive pain	Hydration, analgesics (paracetamol, non-steroidal anti-inflammatory drugs, opioids)
Leg	Leg ulcers	Wound care, compression bandages
Infections	Sepsis, meningitis	Antibiotics
Respiratory	Acute chest syndrome	Hydration, analgesics, respiratory support, antibiotics, bronchodilators, transfusion
Nervous	Ischemic stroke	Resuscitation and stabilisation, hydration, transfusion
	Haemorrhagic stroke	Resuscitation and stabilisation, neurosurgery intervention
Bone	Dactylitis	Hydration, analgesics
	Avascular necrosis	Hydration, analgesics, physiotherapy, crutch-weight bearing, core decompression, arthroplasty
	Osteomyelitis	Antibiotics, operative debridement
Liver	Pigmented gall stones	Cholecystectomy
Kidney	Sickle nephropathy	Avoidance of nephrotoxic drugs, ACE inhibitors, dialysis, renal transplantation
Eyes	Retinopathy	Laser photocoagulation

Allogenic haematopoietic stem cell (HSC) transplantation is the only available cure for sickle cell disease at present. It should be considered in patients with recurrent vaso-occlusive complications who have HLA-matched unaffected sibling donors. Common complications of HSC transplantation are graft failure and graft versus host disease. The overall survival following HSC transplantation is approximately 90% however, lack of HLA-matched family donors is a limiting factor in most patients.

Prognosis

Survival and prognosis of children with SCD have markedly increased over the last decades due to improvements in immunization, antibiotics, use of hydroxyurea and prevention and treatment of disease complications. However, even with the best of care, life expectancy is reduced by approximately 30 years compared to non-sickle cell individuals. Common causes of death are infection, acute chest syndrome, pulmonary hypertension and renal failure.

RECENT ADVANCES

During recent years, significant advances have been made in the development of simple, rapid, reliable and inexpensive point-of-care diagnostic tests for SCD. The techniques that are studied include, paper-based tests that quantify sickle haemoglobin, a density-based rapid test using aqueous multiphase systems and lateral flow immunoassays.

Assessment of blood velocity in the terminal portion of the internal carotid and proximal portion of the middle cerebral artery using transcranial ultrasound is increasingly being used as a reliable predictor of stroke in children with SCD. Maximum time-averaged mean velocity >200cm/s is associated with a high risk of stroke, which can be effectively prevented by starting chronic transfusion therapy in these patients.

Gene therapy with *ex-vivo* transduction of anti-sickling β-globin gene (e.g., AT87Q, AS3) to the patient's own HSCs using lentiviral vectors followed by autologous transplantation after myeloablation has been used in clinical trials. Targeted mutation of γ-globin suppressor genes (e.g., *BCL11A*) by *ex-vivo* genome editing of patient's own HSCs to upregulate γ-globin and HbF have also shown promising results. This approach will also require the infusion of genome corrected autologous HSCs back to patients after myeloablation.

REFERENCES

George, Alex, Michael R DeBaun, and Malcolm R DeBaun. 2019. Acute and chronic bone complications of sickle cell disease. In *UpToDate*, edited by Donald H Mahoney, William A Phillips and Elliott P Vichinsky.

Ghiaccio, V., M. Chappell, S. Rivella, and L. Breda. 2019. "Gene Therapy for Beta-Hemoglobinopathies: Milestones, New Therapies and Challenges." *Mol Diagn Ther* 23 (2):173-186. doi: 10.1007/s40291-019-00383-4.

Kato, G. J., F. B. Piel, C. D. Reid, M. H. Gaston, K. Ohene-Frempong, L. Krishnamurti, W. R. Smith, J. A. Panepinto, D. J. Weatherall, F. F. Costa, and E. P. Vichinsky. 2018. "Sickle cell disease." *Nat Rev Dis Primers* 4:18010. doi: 10.1038/nrdp.2018.10.

Meremikwu, M. M., and U. Okomo. 2016. "Sickle cell disease." *BMJ Clin Evid* 2016.

Piel, F. B., M. H. Steinberg, and D. C. Rees. 2017. "Sickle Cell Disease." *N Engl J Med* 376 (16):1561-1573. doi: 10.1056/NEJMra1510865.

Vanderhave, K. L., C. A. Perkins, B. Scannell, and B. K. Brighton. 2018. "Orthopaedic Manifestations of Sickle Cell Disease." *J Am Acad Orthop Surg* 26 (3):94-101. doi: 10.5435/jaaos-d-16-00255.

Ware, R. E., M. de Montalembert, L. Tshilolo, and M. R. Abboud. 2017. "Sickle cell disease." *Lancet* 390 (10091):311-323. doi: 10.1016/s0140-6736(17)30193-9.

Weatherall, D. J. 2010. "The inherited diseases of hemoglobin are an emerging global health burden." *Blood* 115 (22):4331-6. doi: 10.1182/blood-2010-01-251348.

Chapter 6

OTHER MICROCYTIC ANAEMIAS

Sachith Mettananda*

Department of Paediatrics, University of Kelaniya, Ragama, Sri Lanka

In the proceeding chapters, the most common causes of microcytic anaemia - iron deficiency and haemoglobinopathies - were presented in detail. In this chapter, we will focus on other causes of rare microcytic anaemia in children. Most of these disorders are due to inherited genetic mutations of proteins that are involved in the absorption, transportation, utilization and recycling of iron.

CONGENITAL SIDEROBLASTIC ANAEMIA

Congenital sideroblastic anaemias are a group of inherited conditions caused by abnormalities in haem biosynthesis and mitochondrial function leading to pathological accumulation of iron in mitochondria of erythroid

* Corresponding Author's Email: sachith.mettananda@kln.ac.lk.

precursors. These iron-laden mitochondria are arranged in a perinuclear distribution giving rise to an appearance of the characterize 'ring sideroblasts'.

Genetic Basis

Congenital sideroblastic anaemia (CSA) is caused by mutations in several X-linked and autosomal recessively inherited genes. Mutations in the *ALAS2* (that encodes for the erythroid-specific form of 5-aminolevulinate synthase) is the commonest cause of X-linked sideroblastic anaemia whereas mutations in *SLC25A38* (that encodes an erythroid-specific mitochondrial amino acid carrier which transports glycine into mitochondria) and *GLRX5* (that encodes a protein required for the synthesis of iron-sulphur clusters essential for mitochondrial and cytosolic proteins) causes autosomal recessive sideroblastic anaemia.

Clinical Manifestations

Most children with CSA present during childhood; however, some are not diagnosed until adolescence or adulthood due to mildness of features. A majority are asymptomatic and incidentally detected to have pallor or low haemoglobin with unexplained aetiology. There may be a family history of anaemia in autosomal recessive forms. Commonly physical signs are pallor, icterus, moderate splenomegaly with or without hepatomegaly. Some CSAs are part of syndromes which have other associated manifestations like ataxia (*ABCB7* mutation); immunodeficiency, periodic fevers and developmental delay (*TRNT1* mutation); exocrine pancreas insufficiency (Pearson marrow-pancreas syndrome); and myopathy and lactic acidosis (*PUS1, YARS2, MT-ATP6, LARS2* or *NDUFB11* mutations). Iron overload is a frequent complication of sideroblastic anaemia. Some patients have significant iron overload leading to organ dysfunction that includes liver dysfunction and endocrinopathies.

Investigations and Diagnosis

Laboratory features of CSA are low haemoglobin, low MCV, markedly elevated red cell distribution width (approximately 30) and hypochromic microcytic cells mixed with normal red blood cells (RBCs) in the blood film. Some forms will have normal or high MCV. White blood cells and platelets are usually normal. Serum iron concentration, transferrin saturation and ferritin are usually elevated. The bone marrow aspirate shows normoblastic erythroid hyperplasia with poorly haemoglobinized cytoplasm in erythroblasts. The Prussian blue-stained smear reveals the presence of ring sideroblasts which are erythroid precursors with iron-containing granules surrounding the nucleus. Genetic testing by DNA sequencing using leukocytes from peripheral blood is important to identify the genetic mutation and sub-type of sideroblastic anaemia.

Treatment

Most asymptomatic children with mild anaemia will not require treatment. Alternatively, patients who have severe anaemia will need frequent blood transfusions. Some patients with significant iron overload will require iron chelation treatment with deferasirox, desferrioxamine or deferiprone. A subset of patients with X-linked sideroblastic anaemia responds to oral pyridoxine. Splenectomy is considered a relative contraindication; therefore, should be avoided in patients with CSA as it is usually complicated by fatal thromboembolic events. Haematopoietic stem cell transplantation has been effectively used as a cure in patients with transfusion-dependent sideroblastic anaemia.

Iron Refractory Iron Deficiency Anaemia

Iron refractory iron deficiency anaemia (IRIDA) is characterised by severe iron deficiency anaemia which is resistant to standard doses of oral iron. This is due to autosomal recessive mutations of *TMPRSS6* gene which encodes for matriptase-2, a member of type 2 serine protease family which decreases hepcidin synthesis by the liver. Therefore, *TMPRSS6* mutations enhance the hepcidin synthesis, thus inhibits the intestinal iron absorption and release of iron from reticuloendothelial macrophages in the spleen.

Clinical Manifestations

IRIDA is suspected in children with severe iron deficiency who fail to respond to oral iron treatment for adequate dose and duration. Anaemia is not present during the neonatal period and manifests in early childhood. Other supporting features are no history of dietary iron deficiency, malabsorption or chronic blood loss. There may be a family history of anaemia in a sibling.

Investigations and Diagnosis

Laboratory features are similar to those of severe iron deficiency; low haemoglobin (6-9g/dL), MCV, MCH and MCHC in full blood count, hypochromic microcytic RBCs with anisopoikilocytosis in blood film and low plasma iron and transferrin saturation (usually <5%). Serum ferritin is low or normal, and in contrast to iron deficiency, hepcidin will be high. The diagnosis is confirmed by demonstrating mutations of the *TMPRSS6* gene by gene sequencing.

Treatment

Treatment options of IRIDA include longer courses of higher dose oral iron, concomitant administration of iron and ascorbate and parenteral iron. Parenteral iron treatment results in a progressive increase in haemoglobin, however, it rarely normalizes, and the microcytosis and low transferrin saturation persist. Patients with severe anaemia may require blood transfusions.

HEREDITARY HYPOTRANSFERRINEMIA

Hereditary hypotransferrinemia is an autosomal recessive disorder due to mutations in the transferrin (*TF*) gene. It is characterised by microcytic anaemia and paradoxical iron overload in the liver, heart and pancreas. Lack of transferrin reduces the delivery of iron to the bone marrow for haemoglobin synthesis and erythropoiesis; however, high amount of non-transferrin bound iron in the plasma results in parenchymal iron overload. Laboratory features that support the diagnosis are hypochromic microcytic anaemia, very low or absent transferrin levels and liver iron overload. Genetic testing confirms the diagnosis. Experimental therapies include iron chelation therapy, administration of fresh frozen plasma with a view of replacing transferrin and purified apotransferrin infusions.

HEREDITARY ACERULOPLASMINEMIA

Hereditary aceruloplasminemia is an autosomal recessive condition due to defects in the *CP* gene that encodes ceruloplasmin. In this adult-onset disorder, iron transport from macrophages to plasma for RBC production is impaired; instead, iron accumulates in the brain and visceral organs. It results in mild microcytic anaemia which is associated with retinal degeneration, dementia, chorea, ataxia and diabetes. Laboratory haematological features of mild microcytic anaemia, low iron and transferrin saturation in the presence of high ferritin is suggestive of aceruloplasminemia. The diagnosis is confirmed by undetectable levels of serum ceruloplasmin. Experimental therapies include iron chelation therapy to chelate iron from the brain and other organs, vitamin E or zinc sulphate and administration of fresh frozen plasma with a view of replacing ceruloplasmin.

Divalent Metal Transporter 1 Mutations

Extremely rare autosomal recessive mutations of the *SLC11A2* gene that encodes for divalent metal transporter 1 (DMT1) which promotes iron absorption through duodenal enterocyte and iron egress from cytosolic endosomes result in severe microcytic anaemia along with visceral iron overload. These are characterised by microcytic hypochromic anaemia, elevated serum iron and transferrin saturation, moderately high ferritin and liver iron accumulation.

Lead Toxicity

Lead toxicity is another uncommon acquired cause of microcytic anaemia in children. Important sources of lead leading to toxicity are paint dust from lead-painted surfaces, food or beverages stored in lead-soldered cans or lead-glazed pottery, automobile emissions and lead-using industry. Children less than six years are more susceptible to toxicity with lead. Anaemia in lead toxicity is caused by decreased haemoglobin synthesis by the interference of enzymatic steps in the haem biosynthesis pathway and haemolysis. Other clinical manifestations of lead toxicity are neurocognitive deficits, irritability, lethargy, fatigue, abdominal pain, constipation, renal tubular dysfunction, paralysis due to peripheral neuropathy, hearing loss, seizures and encephalopathy. Lead poisoning is diagnosed by an elevated venous blood lead level. Elevated erythrocyte zinc protoporphyrin (greater than 35μg/dL) level also support the diagnosis. The most important aspect in management is identifying and removing the source of lead while chelation with succimer, calcium disodium ethylenediaminetetraacetic acid and dimercaprol is also used.

Copper Deficiency

Copper deficiency is a rare cause of microcytic anaemia. Its deficiency is associated with severe malnutrition, malabsorption, prolonged parenteral feeding without copper supplementation and excess zinc ingestion. Laboratory features are that of sideroblastic anaemia. Treatment is with oral or parenteral supplementation and treatment of the underlying cause.

References

Brissot, P., D. G. Bernard, E. Brissot, O. Loréal, and M. B. Troadec. 2018. "Rare anemias due to genetic iron metabolism defects." *Mutat Res* 777:52-63. doi: 10.1016/j.mrrev.2018.06.003.

De Falco, L., M. Sanchez, L. Silvestri, C. Kannengiesser, M. U. Muckenthaler, A. Iolascon, L. Gouya, C. Camaschella, and C. Beaumont. 2013. "Iron refractory iron deficiency anemia." *Haematologica* 98 (6):845-53. doi: 10.3324/haematol.2012.075515.

Ducamp, S., and M. D. Fleming. 2019. "The molecular genetics of sideroblastic anemia." *Blood* 133 (1):59-69. doi: 10.1182/blood-2018-08-815951.

Harigae, H., and K. Furuyama. 2010. "Hereditary sideroblastic anemia: pathophysiology and gene mutations." *Int J Hematol* 92 (3):425-31. doi: 10.1007/s12185-010-0688-4.

Iolascon, A., L. De Falco, and C. Beaumont. 2009. "Molecular basis of inherited microcytic anemia due to defects in iron acquisition or heme synthesis." *Haematologica* 94 (3):395-408. doi: 10.3324/haematol. 13619.

Long, Z., H. Li, Y. Du, and B. Han. 2018. "Congenital sideroblastic anemia: Advances in gene mutations and pathophysiology." *Gene* 668:182-189. doi: 10.1016/j.gene.2018.05.074.

Piperno, A., and M. Alessio. 2018. "Aceruloplasminemia: Waiting for an Efficient Therapy." *Front Neurosci* 12:903. doi: 10.3389/fnins.2018.00903.

Pippard, M. J. 2017. "Microcytic anaemias in childhood and iron-refractory iron deficiency anaemia." *Br J Haematol* 177 (2):167-168. doi: 10.1111/bjh.14558.

Part 3.
Normocytic Anaemias

Chapter 7

HEREDITARY SPHEROCYTOSIS AND OTHER MEMBRANOPATHIES

Sachith Mettananda** and Tharindi Suriapperuma
Department of Paediatrics, University of Kelaniya, Ragama, Sri Lanka

Membranopathies are a heterogeneous group of inherited haemolytic anaemias that are due to defective red blood cell (RBC) membranes. They are caused by mutations in genes that encode for RBC membrane or cytoskeleton proteins, transmembrane transporters or ion channels. There are two types of membranopathies; disorders that are due to altered structural organisation of RBC membranes (hereditary spherocytosis, hereditary elliptocytosis, hereditary pyropoikilocytosis and Southeast Asian ovalocytosis) and disorders due to altered membrane transport function (overhydrated stomatocytosis, dehydrated stomatocytosis, familial pseudohyperkalaemia and cryohydrocytosis). Out of these, hereditary spherocytosis is the commonest membranopathy.

---

* Corresponding Author's Email: sachith.mettananda@kln.ac.lk.

Hereditary Spherocytosis

Epidemiology

Hereditary spherocytosis is found in most ethnic groups all over the world. The incidence is higher in European countries (approximately 1:2000 to 1:5000) compared to Africa and Asia.

Genetics and inheritance

There are five genes responsible for causation of hereditary spherocytosis. These hereditary spherocytosis-related genes are *ANK1, SPTA1, SPTB, EPB42* and *SLC4A1,* which encode for RBC membrane and cytoskeleton proteins ankyrin-1, α-spectrin, β-spectrin, protein 4.2 and band 3 respectively. These proteins contribute to regulating the shape and membrane stability of RBCs while maintaining their deformation capabilities to traverse through small blood vessels. Mutations in *ANK1* is responsible for nearly half of patients with hereditary spherocytosis. Mutations in more than one hereditary spherocytosis related genes can give rise to the disease in some individuals. Approximately 75% of patents show autosomal dominant inheritance while others either have an autosomal recessive inheritance or *de novo* mutations. Mutations in *ANK1, SPTB* and *SLC4A1* genes typically show autosomal dominant inheritance, whereas mutations in *SPTA1*, *EPB42* and some mutations of *ANK1* are recessively inherited.

Pathophysiology

The primary functions of the RBC membrane are to maintain the osmolarity, mechanical stability and deformability of cells. The red cell membrane, which is composed of a lipid bilayer and transmembrane proteins, is stabilised by attaching to the intracellular cytoskeleton via protein-protein and lipid-protein interactions. Ankyrin is the major protein that is responsible for mechanical coupling of transmembrane proteins to the cytoskeleton through band 3, spectrin and protein 4.2. Spectrin binds with ankyrin and is responsible for maintaining the shape and the reversible deformability of the cell. Band 3 provides cohesion between the RBC membrane and underlying cytoskeletal proteins. It is important in maintaining cellular water content and the prevention of intracellular dehydration.

Genetic mutations that cause hereditary spherocytosis lead to a deficiency of RBC membrane proteins. This results in the reduced vertical association between the cytoskeleton and membrane proteins, which in turn leads to micro-vesiculation and progressive membrane loss of RBC. Loss of membrane reduces the surface area to volume ratio, thus making RBCs spherocytic. Spherocytic cells lack deformability which is essential to circulate through constricted regions of microcirculation. Repeated passage of these spherocytic cells through the spleen leads to further membrane loss which makes them increasingly spherical. This further impairs their passage through the narrow fenestrations of the splenic cords where they are trapped and prematurely removed from circulation through a process of phagocytosis by splenic macrophages.

Clinical Manifestations

Clinical manifestations of hereditary spherocytosis depend on the severity of haemolysis and anaemia, which can vary from mild well-compensated anaemia to severe transfusion-dependent haemolytic anaemia. The disease can manifest at any age. Most severely affected patients can present during fetal life with severe intrauterine anaemia and hydrops fetalis or during the neonatal period.

Clinical manifestations during the neonatal period are due to excessive haemolysis either causing hyperbilirubinemia or anaemia. Hyperbilirubinemia causes neonatal jaundice that can last for several weeks and can be severe enough to require phototherapy or exchange transfusion. Neonates with hereditary spherocytosis are generally not anaemic at birth. Anaemia becomes evident in the second or third week of life and can be severe enough to require blood transfusions during the first year of life.

Older children present with symptoms of anaemia or jaundice; however, a large proportion is asymptomatic and incidentally detected due to low haemoglobin in full blood count and spherocytes in blood films. Splenomegaly is a universal physical sign after infancy. A certain proportion will present following the development of complications. Complications related to hyperbilirubinemia are pigment gall stones and associated cholecystitis and biliary colic. Complications of chronic anaemia include leg ulcers, growth failure, extramedullary erythropoiesis, transfusion-related iron overload and transient aplastic crisis due to infections such as parvovirus B19. Complications related to splenomegaly are hypersplenism and splenic sequestration leading to acute severe anaemia.

Table 7.1. Severity classification of hereditary spherocytosis

	Mild	Moderate	Severe
Inheritance	Autosomal dominant	Autosomal dominant	Autosomal recessive
Proportion of cases	20-30%	60-75%	3-5%
Symptoms	Asymptomatic	Moderate symptoms	Severe symptoms
Haemoglobin	11-15g/dL	8-12g/dL	6-8g/dL
Reticulocytes	3-6%	>6%	>10%
Bilirubin	1-2mg/dL	>2mg/dL	>3mg/dL
Transfusions	No	Occasional	Frequent
Splenectomy	Rarely	Occasionally	Usually

Severity Classification

Hereditary spherocytosis is classified according to the severity of the disease (Table 7.1) into three groups. Mild cases are asymptomatic and have mild anaemia that is well compensated. Approximately 60-75% of patients have moderately severe disease with symptomatic anaemia and reticulocytosis due to partially compensated haemolysis. Patients with severe hereditary spherocytosis require frequent blood transfusions due to significant haemolysis.

Investigations and Diagnosis

Hereditary spherocytosis is non-immune haemolytic anaemia with evidence of spherocytes in the blood film. Basic investigations reveal typical features of haemolysis; low haemoglobin, reticulocytosis, indirect hyperbilirubinaemia, high lactate dehydrogenase and low serum haptoglobin. Direct and indirect Coombs tests are negative. Evaluation of RBC indices will reveal; high MCHC (≥36 g/dL), and normal to low MCV. Peripheral blood film will show spherocytes and reticulocytes; however, up to one-third of neonates with hereditary spherocytosis do not have significant spherocytes in the blood film (Figure 2.5). Therefore, if the child is stable, it is better to delay further investigations until the child is older than six months. The presence of positive family history, typical clinical and laboratory features and spherocytes in the blood film confirms the diagnosis of hereditary spherocytosis; hence, additional investigations are not required in a majority.

Confirmatory tests for hereditary spherocytosis include EMA (eosin-5'-maleimide) binding, osmotic fragility, cryohaemolysis, acidified glycerol lysis and osmotic gradient ektacytometry tests. None of these tests is 100% accurate; therefore, performing more than one test is recommended. EMA binding test is a flow cytometry-based assay which quantifies the eosin-based fluorescent dye that binds to RBC membrane proteins. In patients with hereditary spherocytosis, mean fluorescence is lower than in controls. This test has high sensitivity (93-96%) and specificity (nearly 93-99%) however, false-negative results occur in patients with mild disease, whereas false-positive results are seen in other membranopathies (e.g., hereditary elliptocytosis, hereditary pyropoikilocytosis, Southeast Asian ovalocytosis), congenital dyserythropoietic anaemia (CDA) type II and autoimmune haemolytic anaemia (AIHA).

In the osmotic fragility test, RBCs are incubated in a progressive dilution of hypotonic sodium chloride solutions, and the fraction of haemoglobin released by haemolysis is measured. Spherocytes haemolyse at lower dilutions due to their lower surface area to volume ratio; hence patients with hereditary spherocytosis have increased osmotic fragility. However, this test has low sensitivity and specificity and can become falsely positive in other condition with spherocytes in the blood. Other tests like cryohaemolysis test and acidified glycerol lysis test have higher sensitivities, however, are not widely available. Osmotic gradient ektacytometry is another useful assay, which gives an idea about red cell deformability, however, is not widely available.

Differential Diagnosis

Spherocytes can be seen in the blood film in several other conditions. AIHA shares similar blood film features to hereditary spherocytosis, however, can be differentiated from Coombs test. Other conditions such as liver disease, thermal injury, micro- and macroangiopathic haemolytic anaemias, clostridial sepsis, haemolytic transfusion reactions, severe hypophosphatemia, ABO incompatibility, and poisoning with a snake, spider, and Hymenoptera venoms are associated with spherocytes in the blood film. Hereditary spherocytosis can also be misdiagnosed as CDA type II. Individuals with hereditary spherocytosis have elevated reticulocyte count, but in CDA type II, reticulocyte response is inadequate for the degree of anaemia.

Treatment

Treatment of hereditary spherocytosis is directed at minimizing complications of chronic haemolysis and anaemia. There is no specific treatment for the RBC membrane defect. All patients with moderate to severe disease should be given oral folic acid (1-2mg/day) supplementation to support erythropoiesis. Blood transfusions are indicated during severe haemolysis and aplastic crises due to parvovirus B19 infection; however, regular transfusions are not generally required. Haemoglobin threshold for transfusion depends on the age, symptoms and co-existing comorbidities. Most patients tolerate lower haemoglobin levels (as low as 5g/dL) without transfusions. Hyperbilirubinaemia in the neonate may require phototherapy or exchange transfusion.

Splenectomy decreases the degree of haemolysis and severity of anaemia in patients with hereditary spherocytosis. It is indicated in patients with severe haemolysis or symptomatic splenomegaly. When possible, splenectomy should be delayed until the child is five years to decrease the risk of sepsis caused by encapsulated organisms. Cholecystectomy is indicated in patients with symptomatic gall stones which can be performed simultaneously with splenectomy.

Follow up and Prognosis

Individuals with mild hereditary spherocytosis require at least one annual clinic visit, whereas patients with severe disease need more frequent monitoring. During follow up growth, symptoms of anaemia and haemoglobin should be monitored. Parents should be well educated about the disease, symptoms of anaemia, complications, the risk of transient aplastic crisis and when to seek early medical advice.

Recent Advances

The most significant advance in the field of red cell membranopathies is the discovery of genes and genetic mutations responsible for various diseases. With the identification of specific genetic mutations, mutation testing panels that uses DNA next-generation sequencing techniques have been developed. This will help to reduce the cost and make diagnoses precisely.

HEREDITARY ELLIPTOCYTOSIS

Hereditary elliptocytosis is an autosomal dominant disease found in all ethnic groups, however, is particularly common in West Africa. Mutations in α-spectrin are responsible for nearly 65% of patients, while mutations in the β-spectrin account for 30%. These mutations cause reduced membrane mechanical stability that results in the progressive transformation of discoid RBCs to elliptocytes and red cell fragmentation. These fragmented RBCs are removed from the circulation by spleen resulting in anaemia.

Hereditary elliptocytosis has a wide phenotypic variation ranging from asymptomatic disease to severe anaemia. Elliptocytes in the blood film is characteristic (Figure 2.5). In moderate to severe disease, blood films will also show fragmented cells. Patients with severe disease will benefit from splenectomy, which will reduce the severity of the anaemia by increasing the life span of fragmented cells.

HEREDITARY PYROPOIKILOCYTOSIS

Hereditary pyropoikilocytosis is a subtype of hereditary elliptocytosis which is characterized by poikilocytes, spherocytes, fragmented RBCs and extreme microcytosis (MCV 30-50fL) in the blood film. It shows autosomal recessive inheritance pattern. These patients have severe haemolysis and significant splenomegaly, therefore, require frequent blood transfusions and splenectomy.

SOUTHEAST ASIAN OVALOCYTOSIS

Southeast Asian ovalocytosis is an autosomal dominant condition due to a structural abnormality in RBC membrane causing changes in the erythrocyte membrane permeability. Most patients are asymptomatic. Ovalocytes with one or more transverse slits in blood film is characteristic.

HEREDITARY STOMATOCYTOSIS

There are two types of hereditary stomatocytosis; overhydrated stomatocytosis and dehydrated stomatocytosis or hereditary xerocytosis. Overhydrated stomatocytosis is due to defective permeability of red cell membrane leading to excess intracellular sodium leading to an increase in cellular water content causing overhydration. RBCs become less deformable, thus are removed from the circulation by spleen. Clinical features are mild to moderate haemolytic anaemia and reticulocytosis. MCV is increased, and MCHC is low. Blood film evidence of stomatocytes is a characteristic feature of this disease. There is no specific treatment, and splenectomy is not beneficial.

Hereditary xerocytosis is a dominantly inherited disorder with an inability to maintain normal intracellular sodium and potassium. The disruption in volume homeostasis will make the cells lose water and lead to dehydration and increased cell membrane rigidity. Individuals with hereditary xerocytosis have mild to moderate haemolytic anaemia which could sometimes be asymptomatic. MCV is normal or high, whereas MCHC is increased. Peripheral blood film is normal except for a few stomatocytes, target cells and contracted red cells. No specific treatment is available; splenectomy is not recommended.

References

Andolfo, I., R. Russo, A. Gambale, and A. Iolascon. 2016. "New insights on hereditary erythrocyte membrane defects." *Haematologica* 101 (11):1284-1294. doi: 10.3324/haematol.2016.142463.

Bolton-Maggs, P. H., J. C. Langer, A. Iolascon, P. Tittensor, M. J. King, and Haematology General Haematology Task Force of the British Committee for Standards in. 2012. "Guidelines for the diagnosis and management of hereditary spherocytosis--2011 update." *Br J Haematol* 156 (1):37-49. doi: 10.1111/j.1365-2141.2011.08921.x.

Da Costa, L., J. Galimand, O. Fenneteau, and N. Mohandas. 2013. "Hereditary spherocytosis, elliptocytosis, and other red cell membrane disorders." *Blood Rev* 27 (4):167-78. doi: 10.1016/j.blre.2013.04.003.

Gallagher, P. G. 2017. "Disorders of erythrocyte hydration." *Blood* 130 (25):2699-2708. doi: 10.1182/blood-2017-04-590810.

He, B. J., L. Liao, Z. F. Deng, Y. F. Tao, Y. C. Xu, and F. Q. Lin. 2018. "Molecular Genetic Mechanisms of Hereditary Spherocytosis: Current Perspectives." *Acta Haematol* 139 (1):60-66. doi: 10.1159/000486229.

Iolascon, A., I. Andolfo, and R. Russo. 2019. "Advances in understanding the pathogenesis of red cell membrane disorders." *Br J Haematol* 187 (1):13-24. doi: 10.1111/bjh.16126.

Mohandas, N. 2018. "Inherited hemolytic anemia: a possessive beginner's guide." *Hematology Am Soc Hematol Educ Program* 2018 (1):377-381. doi: 10.1182/asheducation-2018.1.377.

Narla, J., and N. Mohandas. 2017. "Red cell membrane disorders." *Int J Lab Hematol* 39 Suppl 1:47-52. doi: 10.1111/ijlh.12657.

Zamora, E. A., and C. A. Schaefer. 2020. "Hereditary Spherocytosis." In *StatPearls*. Treasure Island (FL): StatPearls Publishing Copyright © 2020, StatPearls Publishing LLC.

Chapter 8

GLUCOSE-6-PHOSPHATE DEHYDROGENASE DEFICIENCY AND OTHER RED CELL ENZYMOPATHIES

Duantida Songdej[1,*] and Tharindi Suriapperuma[2]
[1]Ramathibodi Hospital of Mahidol University, Bangkok, Thailand
[2]Department of Paediatrics, University of Kelaniya, Ragama, Sri Lanka

Mature human red blood cells (RBCs) do not contain nuclei or endoplasmic reticula. Therefore, all metabolic activities depend upon two major glucose metabolic pathways (Figure 8.1). They are;

1. Embden-Meyerhof pathway: This is an anaerobic glycolytic process, which produces two molecules of adenosine triphosphate (ATP) at the end to be utilized as an energy source for RBCs. This pathway is driven by kinase group of enzymes which include three

---

* Corresponding Author's Email: duantida.son@mahidol.ac.th.

major rate-limiting step kinases; phosphofructokinase, hexokinase and pyruvate kinase.

2. Hexose monophosphate shunt: Glucose-6-phosphate dehydrogenase (G6PD) which converts glucose-6-phosphate to 6-phosphogluconolactone is the rate-limiting step enzyme of this pathway. During this step, nicotinamide adenine dinucleotide phosphate (NADP) is converted to the reduced form of NADP (i.e. NADPH). NADPH protects cells from oxidative stress by maintaining reduced glutathione in RBCs.

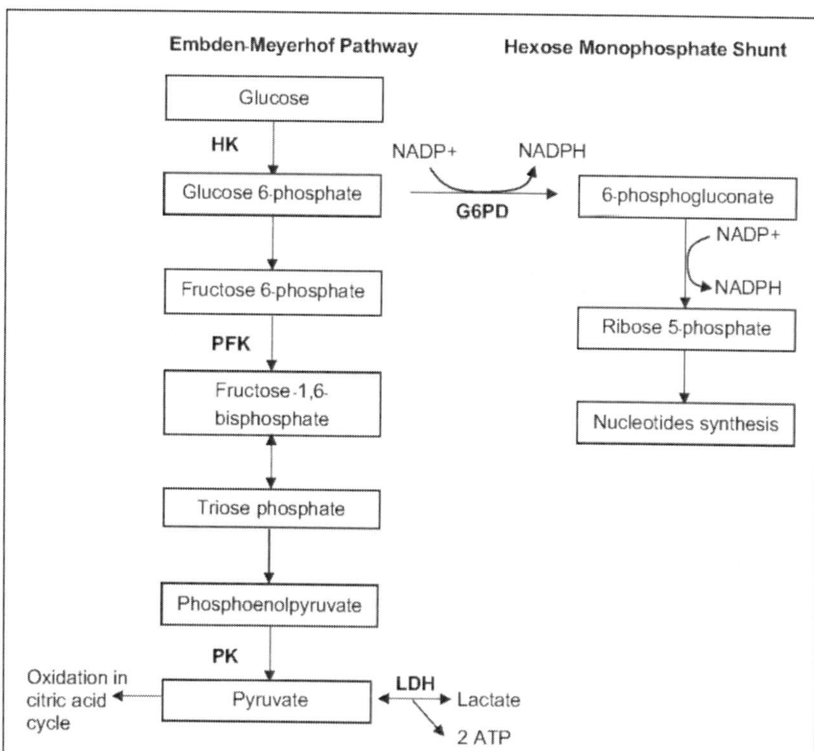

Figure 8.1. Glucose metabolism in red blood cells. In red blood cells, glucose is metabolized via the Embden-Meyerhof pathway (left panel) and Hexose Monophosphate Shunt (right panel). Bolded alphabets indicate rate-limiting step enzymes. HK = hexokinase, PFK = phosphofructokinase, PK = pyruvate kinase, LDH = lactase dehydrogenase and G6PD = glucose-6-phosphate dehydrogenase.

In this chapter, the two most prevalent red cell enzymopathies, G6PD and pyruvate kinase deficiencies will be described.

Glucose-6-Phosphate Dehydrogenase Deficiency

Epidemiology

G6PD deficiency is the most common red cell enzymopathy affecting over 400 million people worldwide. It is found in all continents, but higher prevalence is reported in Africa, southern Europe and Asia with the highest prevalence of 60-70% reported among Kurdish Jews. The geographic distribution of G6PD deficiency is similar to the distribution of malaria, leading to a hypothesis that those affected by G6DP deficiency are protected from malaria infection.

Genetics and Inheritance

G6PD gene is located at the long arm of the X chromosome (band Xq28) near the telomeric region, which is recognized as a hot spot in the human genome. More than 180 genetic mutations of the *G6PD* gene which show X-linked recessive inheritance have been reported thus far. Males are hemizygous; therefore, if their X chromosome is carrying a *G6PD* gene mutation, they manifest features of G6PD deficiency. Females who carry *G6PD* mutation in one of their X chromosomes are heterozygous carriers. The phenotype of these females could vary from normal G6PD enzyme levels to intermediate or gross deficiency of G6PD enzymes depending on the presence of X-chromosome mosaicism and X-inactivation. Females who are homozygous for *G6PD* gene mutation show phenotype of G6PD deficiency.

Pathophysiology

The main role of G6PD enzyme is to synthesize NADPH to regenerate and maintain reduced glutathione. Reduced glutathione is protective against oxidative stress created by certain drugs, acute infections and food. When G6PD deficient RBCs are exposed to oxidants, they become depleted of reduced glutathione resulting in accumulation of reactive oxygen species leading to acute intravascular haemolysis. Glutathione depletion also leads to oxidation of sulfhydryl containing proteins, including haemoglobin. This leads to the production of methaemoglobin and denatured globin, which can be visualized as insoluble masses known as 'Heinz bodies' attached to RBC membranes when stained with supravital stain. Due to cross-bonding of denatured haemoglobin, free flow of haemoglobin in the cytosol is lost. Moreover, oxidation of sulfhydryl groups of RBC membrane proteins leads to the accumulation of polypeptide aggregates due to disulphide bond formation between spectrin dimers and other proteins. The ultimate effect is that reduced glutathione deficient RBCs become rigid and lack the ability of deformation. Less deformable RBCs are trapped in the microcirculation and prematurely removed by the reticuloendothelial macrophages in the spleen, liver and marrow resulting in extravascular haemolysis. Extravascular haemolysis is more common in individuals with class I variants, who suffer from chronic non-spherocytic haemolytic anaemia.

Classification

According to the residual activity of G6PD enzyme and the degree of haemolysis, G6PD deficiency is classified into five classes by the World Health Organization (WHO) (Table 8.1).

Table 8.1. Classification of G6PD deficiency

	Residual G6PD activity	Degree of haemolysis
Class I	Severely deficient (<10% residual activity)	Chronic haemolytic anaemia
Class II	Severely deficient (<10% residual activity)	Intermittent haemolysis associated with infection, drugs or chemicals
Class III	Moderately deficient (10-60% residual activity)	Intermittent haemolysis associated with infection, drugs or chemicals
Class IV	Normal activity (60-100% activity)	No haemolysis
Class V	More than twice normal activity	No haemolysis

A majority of *G6PD* mutations are associated with WHO class II and III. Some *G6PD* variants are more common in specific parts of the world. For example, the *G6PD* Mediterranean variant which is associated with WHO class II is the commonest variant in the Mediterranean and the Middle East. *G6PD* A^- variant, which is a class III variant, is predominantly reported in African ancestry. Affected individuals often present with mild to moderate acute intravascular haemolysis. Reticulocytes in individuals with G6PD A- variant demonstrate normal enzyme activity. *G6PD* variants that are more common among Asians include *G6PD* Canton, *G6PD* Kaiping, *G6PD* Gaohe and *G6PD* Mahidol. These variants are associated with WHO Class II or III. There is no clinical significance of G6PD deficiency of WHO class IV and V.

Clinical Manifestations

Disease severity varies with the degree of G6PD enzyme deficiency. Majority of G6PD deficient individuals are asymptomatic and manifest as acute haemolytic anaemia when exposed to oxidant stress due to drugs, acute infections, illnesses, or foods. Drugs that can induce acute intravascular haemolysis in affected individuals are listed in Table 8.2. The clinical presentation typically includes jaundice, pallor and dark urine indicating haemoglobinuria, 2-4 days after the exposure to oxidant stress.

Haemolytic anaemia may last for 7-8 days which then resolve spontaneously. Infections which are associated with acute haemolysis in G6PD deficient individuals include viral hepatitis (hepatitis A and B), cytomegalovirus, dengue, pneumonia and typhoid fever. Some of the affected individuals manifest features of "favism" following ingestion of fresh fava bean. Favism occurs most often in individuals with certain G6PD deficiency variants (*G6PD* Mediterranean and G6PD Canton) mostly from Italy, Greece, North Africa, the Middle East and Asia. It is less common in Africans and African Americans. This usually occurs between 1-5 years of age. Acute severe haemolytic anaemia occurs within 24 hours of ingestion, and this may lead to massive haemoglobinuria and precipitating haemoglobin casts resulting in acute kidney injury.

Table 8.2. Drugs associated with acute haemolysis in G6PD deficiency

Drugs with a definite association	Drugs with a possible association	Drugs with a doubtful association
Primaquine	Chloroquine	Mepacrine
Pamaquine	Sulfadimidine	Quinine
Sulphanilamide	Sulfasalazine	Aldesulfone
Sulfacetamide	Glibenclamide	Sulfadiazine
Sulphapyridine	Aspirin	Sulfafurazole
Sulfamethoxazole	Ciprofloxacin	Paracetamol
Dapsone	Chloramphenicol	Phenacetin
Nitrofurantoin	Vitamin K analogues	Aminosalicylic acid
Acetanilide	Ascorbic acid	Doxorubicin
Nalidixic acid	Mesalazine	Probenecid
Niridazole	Acalypha indica extract	Dimercaprol
Methylthionium		
Phenazopyridine		
Co-trimoxazole		
2,4,6-trinitrotoluene		
Naphthalene		

Neonates with G6PD deficiency due to class II and III variants present with jaundice. For example, 22% of male and 10% of female Thai neonates who had neonatal jaundice were found to have G6PD deficiency. These neonates tend to develop jaundice in 1-4 days of life. Individuals with

G6PD class I variants typically present with chronic non-spherocytic haemolytic anaemia even in the absence of oxidative stress. Even though the term 'non-spherocytic' is commonly used, peripheral blood film of these patients may contain few spherocytes. Most of these individuals maintain haemoglobin around 8-10g/dL along with reticulocytosis of 10-15%. Intermittent jaundice is a common feature, though pallor and splenomegaly are uncommon. Gall stones are a possible complication.

Investigations and Diagnosis

Screening for G6PD deficiency should be performed in the following clinical situations;

1. Individuals with acute haemolytic anaemia following ingestion of offending drugs;
2. Family history of neonatal jaundice, splenomegaly or gall stones;
3. Every neonate with significant neonatal jaundice;
4. Individuals living in malaria-endemic areas and requiring anti-malarial drugs.

For those who present with acute haemolysis, initial investigations include evidence to support haemolytic anaemia. These are low haemoglobin, increased reticulocyte count, indirect hyperbilirubinaemia and reduced haptoglobin. Direct Coombs test is negative. Confirmation of G6PD deficiency is made by performing screening and diagnostic tests in a stepwise manner. Screening tests for G6PD deficiency are:

1. Peripheral blood smear: During an acute haemolytic episode, peripheral blood film shows characteristic features including blister cells, bite cells, basket cells, eccentrocytes or contracted haemoglobin red blood cells (Figure 2.5). These features show haemoglobin leakage from red blood cells;

2. Heinz bodies: Heinz bodies can be visualized as a dark spot at a rim of RBC by supravital staining of the blood smears. This is resulted from denatured haemoglobin after exposing to oxidative stress;
3. Fluorescent spot test: Fluorescent spot test is a semiquantitative assay which is most often used for mass screening of G6PD deficiency in malaria-endemic areas. This test is easy to perform, cheap and rapid, therefore widely used in hospital settings as well. It has over 95% sensitivity and is specific to detect G6PD deficient individuals who are having residual enzyme activity <30%.

There are two types of diagnostic tests to confirm G6PD deficiency. These are;

1. G6PD activity assay: This method indirectly quantifies residual G6PD enzyme activity by measuring newly generated NADPH, following a mix of sample hemolysate, glucose-6-phosphate and NADP using spectrophotometry;
2. G6PD molecular analysis: This can be performed using Sanger sequencing, polymerase chain reaction (PCR)-restriction enzyme-based method or multiplex amplification refractory mutation system-PCR (ARMS-PCR).

Both fluorescent spot test and G6PD activity assay could become falsely negative in an acute episode of haemolysis. During haemolysis, RBCs which are deficient in G6PD enzyme are removed from the circulation. However, younger RBCs and reticulocytes, which has a higher amount of G6PD enzyme increases. Therefore, the assays will over-estimate the amount of G6PD enzyme in normal red blood cells giving false negative results. If strong clinical suspicion remains, it is generally recommended to repeat the assays three months after resolution of haemolysis. Newborn screening using the fluorescent spot test is offered in populations where G6PD deficiency is highly prevalent. Prenatal testing is not commonly done.

Differential Diagnosis

Many inherited and acquired haemolytic anaemias form the differential diagnosis of G6PD deficiency. Inherited haemolytic anaemias such as other enzymopathies (e.g., pyruvate kinase deficiency), haemoglobin-pathies (e.g., thalassaemia syndromes) and membranopathies (eg, hereditary spherocytosis) share similar clinical features including chronic haemolysis (similar to that found in *G6PD* variants class I) and acute haemolytic episodes following stress. Acquired haemolytic anaemias of immune or non-immune aetiology also share similar clinical features. Direct and indirect Coombs tests must be performed to exclude autoimmune, alloimmune and isoimmune haemolytic anaemias. Screening tests and diagnostic tests will help to differentiate G6PD deficiency from other haemolytic anaemias.

Treatment

The mainstay in the management of G6PD deficiency is preventing exposure of oxidants to erythrocytes, that are known to trigger haemolysis. G6PD deficient neonates with jaundice are managed similar to neonatal jaundice from other causes. These include phototherapy or exchange transfusion as required to prevent bilirubin encephalopathy.

Once acute haemolysis occurs, avoid further exposure to the offending agents. Most acute haemolytic episodes are short-lasting and can be managed without blood transfusions. Blood transfusions are required only if individuals present with symptomatic anaemia with fatigue, dizziness, haemic murmur or haemodynamic instability. Aggressive hydration is required to prevent the formation of haemoglobin casts and acute kidney injury following acute intravascular haemolysis.

Affected individuals with chronic haemolytic anaemia do not always require regular blood transfusions. Most of them are well compensated. Very few individuals will develop transfusion-dependent anaemia leading to iron overload requiring iron chelation. Antioxidants such as vitamin E and selenium had been tried, but no proven benefit has been established. These individuals can be prescribed on routine folic acid supplementation, but patients with infrequent episodes of haemolysis do not require regular supplementation. Splenectomy has no benefit in G6PD deficiency.

Patient Education

Parents of children with G6PD deficiency should be informed that certain food, drugs and infections/illnesses can trigger acute haemolytic episodes. Symptoms of intravascular haemolysis such as pallor, jaundice and dark urine should be made aware to affected individuals. They should carry a card with the diagnosis and list of drugs and food to be avoided. They should be told to disclose their G6PD deficient status in every medical encounter or show the G6PD identification card.

Follow Up and Prognosis

G6PD deficient individuals generally have excellent prognosis as most of them are asymptomatic throughout life. Patients with infrequent episodes of acute haemolysis do not need regular visits to the clinic. Individuals with chronic haemolysis need regular follow up to assess the degree of anaemia and haemolysis. Any triggering factor such as infections, foods and medications can worsen pre-existing anaemia. They are recommended to have regular folic acid supplementation. Iron overload is not common in G6PD deficiency unless they are transfusion-dependent, which is very rare.

Recent Advances

During the last few years, advances had been in the aspect of widening the understanding of the disease by identifying 31 new gene mutations. The localization of these mutations was done by solving the structure of the G6PD protein and using bioinformatics tools. Most of the variants belong to class I. Identification of new mutations may improve the understanding of the disease and will open new treatment options in the future.

PYRUVATE KINASE DEFICIENCY

Pyruvate kinase deficiency is extremely rare, though it is considered as the second commonest enzymopathy and the commonest enzymopathy leading to chronic haemolysis. Prevalence in the white population is approximately 1:20,000. Mutations in the *PKLR* gene which encode for pyruvate kinase enzyme is inherited in an autosomal recessive fashion. More than 300 *PKLR* mutations have been identified to date. Pyruvate kinase is the terminal enzyme in glycolysis, and this process helps cells to produce energy in the form of ATP (Figure 8.1). The deficiency of pyruvate kinase enzyme leads to instability of electrochemical gradient of RBCs. This results in a shorter lifespan of mature RBCs and reticulocytes and deformed red cell membrane will be destroyed by spleen (extravascular haemolysis).

Clinical Manifestations

Typical clinical features of pyruvate kinase deficiency are anaemia and symptoms of extravascular haemolysis. There is a wide range of clinical severity from fetal hydrops to asymptomatic anaemia. A vast majority (90%) of affected babies have significant neonatal jaundice requiring phototherapy or exchange transfusion. Eighty per cent of patients have splenomegaly, and 40-70% develop gall stones. However, patients with pyruvate kinase deficiency are more tolerant to anaemia, as compared to those with other chronic haemolytic anaemias. This is because pyruvate kinase deficiency leads to an increased level of red cell 2,3-diphosphoglycerate, which in turn results in a rightward shift of oxy-haemoglobin dissociation curve. Acute haemolysis may occur on top of chronic haemolysis following stress.

Investigations and Diagnosis

The peripheral blood film of affected patients is nonspecific with some echinocytes (burr cells), adipocytes or poikilocytes. Some individuals have normal RBC morphology. Diagnosis is established by measuring pyruvate kinase activity in RBCs using spectrophotometry. Identification of *PKLR* gene mutation is also recommended in parallel with the measurement of enzyme activity.

Treatment

In patients with symptomatic anaemia, bone change and growth restriction, regular blood transfusions are recommended. Folic acid supplementation and iron chelation are important measures in the management of this group of patients. There is evidence that splenectomy improves the average baseline haemoglobin level by 1.6g/dL. However, this procedure should be reserved for patients with severe transfusion-dependent anaemia due to post-splenectomy complications, including increased risk of encapsulated bacterial infection and thrombotic events.

Recent Advances

Several new treatment strategies are under investigation for pyruvate kinase deficiency. Allogeneic haematopoietic cell transplantation is being evaluated as a potential treatment option for patients who require chronic transfusions even after splenectomy. Being a monogenic disorder, pyruvate kinase deficiency is more likely to be cured by gene therapy. Still, there are no clinical trials on gene therapy or gene editing however, *in vivo* studies in mouse models are ongoing. Also, an oral medication which can activate pyruvate kinase enzyme in erythrocytes (Mitapivat) is under research.

REFERENCES

Agarwal, A. M., and A. Rets. 2020. "Laboratory approach to investigation of anemia with a focus on pyruvate kinase deficiency." *Int J Lab Hematol* 42 Suppl 1:107-112. doi: 10.1111/ijlh.13200.

Banyatsuppasin, W., S. Jindadamrongwech, A. Limrungsikul, and P. Butthep. 2017. "Prevalence of Thalassemia and Glucose-6-Phosphate Dehydrogenase Deficiency in Newborns and Adults at the Ramathibodi Hospital, Bangkok, Thailand." *Hemoglobin* 41 (4-6):260-266. doi: 10. 1080/03630269.2017.1402026.

Cappellini, M. D., and G. Fiorelli. 2008. "Glucose-6-phosphate dehydrogenase deficiency." *Lancet* 371 (9606):64-74. doi: 10.1016/s0140-6736(08)60073-2.

Charoenkwan, P., W. Tantiprabha, S. Sirichotiyakul, A. Phusua, and T. Sanguansermsri. 2014. "Prevalence and molecular characterization of glucose-6-phosphate dehydrogenase deficiency in northern Thailand." *Southeast Asian J Trop Med Public Health* 45 (1):187-93.

Grace, R. F., P. Bianchi, E. J. van Beers, S. W. Eber, B. Glader, H. M. Yaish, J. M. Despotovic, J. A. Rothman, M. Sharma, M. M. McNaull, E. Fermo, K. Lezon-Geyda, D. H. Morton, E. J. Neufeld, S. Chonat, N. Kollmar, C. M. Knoll, K. Kuo, J. L. Kwiatkowski, D. Pospíšilová, Y. D. Pastore, A. A. Thompson, P. E. Newburger, Y. Ravindranath, W. C. Wang, M. W. Wlodarski, H. Wang, S. Holzhauer, V. R. Breakey, J. Kunz, S. Sheth, M. J. Rose, H. A. Bradeen, N. Neu, D. Guo, H. Al-Sayegh, W. B. London, P. G. Gallagher, A. Zanella, and W. Barcellini. 2018. "Clinical spectrum of pyruvate kinase deficiency: data from the Pyruvate Kinase Deficiency Natural History Study." *Blood* 131 (20):2183-2192. doi: 10.1182/blood-2017-10-810796.

Grace, R. F., D. Mark Layton, and W. Barcellini. 2019. "How we manage patients with pyruvate kinase deficiency." *Br J Haematol* 184 (5):721-734. doi: 10.1111/bjh.15758.

Nuchprayoon, I., S. Sanpavat, and S. Nuchprayoon. 2002. "Glucose-6-phosphate dehydrogenase (G6PD) mutations in Thailand: G6PD Viangchan (871G>A) is the most common deficiency variant in the Thai population." *Hum Mutat* 19 (2):185. doi: 10.1002/humu.9010.

Sedano, I. B., B. Rothlisberger, G. Deleze, C. Ottiger, M. A. Panchard, A. Spahr, M. Hergersberg, W. Burgi, and A. Huber. 2004. "PK Aarau: first homozygous nonsense mutation causing pyruvate kinase deficiency." *Br J Haematol* 127 (3):364-6. doi: 10.1111/j.1365-2141.2004.05209.x.

Chapter 9

AUTOIMMUNE HAEMOLYTIC ANAEMIA

Duantida Songdej[1,*] and Tharindi Suriapperuma[2]
[1]Ramathibodi Hospital of Mahidol University, Bangkok, Thailand
[2]Department of Paediatrics, University of Kelaniya, Ragama, Sri Lanka

Autoimmune haemolytic anaemia (AIHA) is characterized by premature destruction of erythrocytes by autoantibodies acting against one's own red blood cell (RBC) antigens. The hallmark of this disorder is a positive direct Coombs test (also referred to as direct antiglobulin test, DAT) from which the causative immune complexes can be sub-identified into immunoglobulin (Ig) G, IgM and complement C3d. The disease manifestations and treatment options vary, depending on the aetiology of AIHA and DAT profile.

EPIDEMIOLOGY

The estimated incidence of AIHA in children is 0.8-1.25 per 100,000. It affects all populations and age groups worldwide. The incidence,

[*] Corresponding Author's Email: duantida.son@mahidol.ac.th.

however, increases with age. Among children, it commonly occurs 2-3 weeks following infections, whereas in adult, it is reported following usage of medication, leukaemia and autoimmune diseases in addition to infection.

Genetics and Inheritance

There is no identified genetic predisposition or inheritance pattern for AIHA.

Pathophysiology

AIHA is caused by the production of autoantibodies or immune complexes that react against RBC antigens. These antibodies could be immunoglobulins of any type; however, they are commonly of IgG or IgM type and rarely of IgA type. Apart from immunoglobulins, complement proteins also play a significant role in the pathogenesis of AIHA, which ultimately results in premature destruction of erythrocytes; either extravascular or intravascular. Autoantibodies of IgG type react with protein antigens in the erythrocyte surface optimally at normal body temperature (37^0C). Therefore, these antibodies are called 'warm agglutinins'; nonetheless, they hardly play a role in the RBC agglutination. In contrast, IgM antibodies bind to polysaccharide antigens on the erythrocyte surface at lower temperatures with maximum binding occurring around 4°C. Consequently, these antibodies are known as 'cold agglutinins' which often contribute to RBC agglutination.

Classification

AIHA is classified into three main groups, based on the optimal temperature at which autoantibodies bind to erythrocyte antigens *in vivo* (thermal reactivity); Warm reactive AIHA, cold agglutinin disease and paroxysmal cold haemoglobinuria.

- Warm reactive AIHA is the most common type of AIHA seen in children, accounting for 60-90% of patients. Warm reactive autoantibodies which are typically of IgG type bind to RBC antigens at 37°C. Fc portions of IgG are subsequently bound to Fc receptors on macrophages, leading to phagocytosis and extravascular haemolysis. This event is primarily taking place in the spleen. However, intravascular haemolysis is also recognized in a minority. Some patients with warm reactive AIHA have C3d positivity with or without IgG.
- Cold agglutinin disease (CAD) is uncommon during childhood and accounts for approximately 10% of cases. Characteristic IgM autoantibodies bind to RBC antigens at colder temperatures (maximum at 4°C). The binding of these antibodies occurs primarily at I/i antigen and less commonly at Pr antigen of RBCs leading to fixation of complement. The DAT profile is positive for C3d and can be weakly positive for IgG. The haemolysis occurs both intravascularly and extravascularly. The intravascular haemolysis is mediated by complement proteins, whereas extravascular haemolysis is an immune-mediated process. Primary CAD or idiopathic CAD is rare. In most patients, CAD is secondary to infections such as *Mycoplasma pneumoniae*, Epstein-Barr virus and cytomegalovirus, autoimmune disorders including systemic lupus erythematosus or aggressive lymphoma.
- Paroxysmal cold haemoglobinuria (PCH) is caused by Donath-Landsteiner antibodies, which are of IgG type that reacts against the P antigen of erythrocytes. It is a self-limiting disease occurring almost exclusively in children below 18 years and often triggered by infection, including viruses and syphilis. Donath-Landsteiner autoantibodies bind to RBCs and fix complement protein C1 at colder temperatures. However, complement activation leading to intravascular haemolysis occurs at a core temperature of 37°C. Due

to this difference, these antibodies are frequently known as 'biphasic haemolysins'.

- Mixed AIHA is characterised by RBC destruction caused by both warm IgG and cold IgM antibodies. DAT profile is positive for both IgG and C3d.

AIHA is also divided into two groups as primary and secondary AIHA based on the underlying disease process.

- Primary AIHA or Idiopathic AIHA occurs without an underlying systemic illness. Most primary AIHAs are caused by warm reactive autoantibodies, and this group comprises of 40-50% of paediatric patients.
- Secondary AIHA occurs following a recognizable underlying systemic illness. The majority of secondary AIHAs are also caused by warm reactive autoantibodies; however, CAD is recognized when triggered by infective aetiologies, including *Mycoplasma pneumoniae*, Epstein-Barr virus and cytomegalovirus. Causes of secondary warm AIHA include autoimmune and connective tissue disorders (e.g., systemic lupus erythematosus), immune deficiency disorders (e.g., common variable immune deficiency), malignancy (e.g., lymphoma and chronic myeloid leukaemia), HIV infection, other viral infections and bone marrow or solid organ transplantation.

Evans syndrome is a special variant of AIHA associated with two or more immune-mediated cytopenias; the majority have AIHA and immune thrombocytopenia. Approximately 50% of individuals affected with Evans syndrome have underlying systemic disorders such as systemic lupus erythematosus, common variable immune deficiency or autoimmune lymphoreticular disorder.

Drug-related immune haemolysis is responsible for a small proportion of patients with AIHA. Two types of reactions between drugs and erythrocytes are responsible for haemolysis. Firstly, RBC antigens can be altered by various medications leading to the production of antibodies (IgG or IgM) against altered antigens which can then cross-react with unaltered antigens. Secondly, drugs can get attached to a part of the antigen present in the RBC surface.

Clinical Manifestations

Most clinical features of AIHA share features of other haemolytic disorders. Symptoms and signs of AIHA depend on the severity of haemolysis and anaemia. These can vary from asymptomatic state due to mild haemolysis to severe life-threatening anaemia due to profound haemolysis. Commonly reported symptoms due to anaemia are dizziness, body weakness and fatigue. Symptoms of haemolysis include yellowish discolouration of the body and dark red or cola colour urine due to haemoglobinuria. Haemoglobinuria suggests intravascular haemolysis. Some individuals present with fever and abdominal pain. Common physical signs of AIHA include pallor, icterus and systolic flow murmurs. Profound anaemia can be complicated by features of heart failure that include tachypnoea, shortness of breath, ankle oedema, tachycardia, cardiomegaly and hepatosplenomegaly. Acrocyanosis, Raynaud's disease, livedo reticularis and cutaneous ulcerations are less common features of AIHA particularly related to CAD. Also, an increased risk of venous thromboembolism is reported to be associated with CAD.

Investigations and Diagnosis

Initial investigations of a suspected patient with AIHA should be directed at establishing the presence of haemolytic anaemia. These include full blood count to confirm anaemia and to determine its severity, serum bilirubin to demonstrate indirect hyperbilirubinaemia, reticulocyte count and percentage to show reticulocytosis and low serum haptoglobin levels.

Serum lactate dehydrogenase and aspartate aminotransferase levels are elevated especially in the presence of intravascular haemolysis. The MCV will be typically normal; however, it can be unexpectedly high due to cold or warm agglutinins resulting in RBC clumps. Reticulocytopenia occurs less commonly if AIHA is associated with parvovirus B19 infection or immune destruction of erythroid precursors. Blood film in AIHA shows normocytic anaemia, polychromatic cells and nucleated RBCs reflecting haemolysis and accelerated erythropoiesis (Figure 2.5). The presence of micro-spherocytes and red cell fragments are more in favour of warm AIHA, whereas CAD is characterized by clumped or agglutinated RBCs.

DAT is positive in most patients with AIHA. However, DAT is not specific and can be positive in other immune-mediated haemolytic diseases including delayed transfusion reaction, drug-induced haemolysis, haemolysis following allogeneic stem cell or solid organ transplantation and haemolytic disease of the newborn. Similarly, DAT can be negative in AIHA in the presence of lower titres of autoantibodies or IgA antibodies. When the clinical suspicion of AIHA is high, and the DAT is negative, gel cards or flow cytometry can be used to detect IgA autoantibodies or warm reactive IgM antibodies. However, these tests have limited availability.

DAT profile is helpful to diagnose the type of AIHA. Most individuals with warm AIHA are positive for anti-IgG alone or both anti-IgG and anti-C3d antibodies. Patients with CAD are positive for anti-C3d antibodies; only a minority will be positive for anti-IgG antibodies, albeit weakly. Patients with PCH are positive for IgG Donath-Landsteiner antibodies.

The diagnosis of warm AIHA is established by biochemical markers of haemolytic anaemia, spherocytes in the blood film and positive DAT for IgG or C3d. CAD is diagnosed by biochemical markers of haemolytic anaemia, characteristic DAT profile and high cold agglutinin titre. Once the diagnosis of AIHA is established, further investigations should be done to evaluate for a secondary cause. These include; antinuclear antibodies, serum immunoglobulin levels and in children with CAD *Mycoplasma pneumoniae* IgM antibodies and Epstein-Barr virus IgM antibodies.

Differential Diagnosis

Nonimmune haemolytic anaemias and non-haemolytic causes of jaundice and dark urine share some clinical and biochemical features of AIHA. Nonimmune haemolytic anaemias such as haemoglobinopathies, membranopathies, enzymopathies and extrinsic causes of haemolysis form the main differential diagnosis. Positive DAT helps to differentiate AIHA from other haemolytic anaemias. Liver disease and disorders of bilirubin metabolism such as Gilbert syndrome can present with jaundice; however, they do not show evidence of haemolysis. Myoglobinuria due to rhabdomyolysis presents with dark colour urine but is not associated with haemolysis or icterus.

Treatment

Severe AIHA with profound haemolysis can pose a medical emergency. These patients should be adequately resuscitated to optimise intravascular volume. The least incompatible blood should be transfused to correct severe life-threatening anaemia. In some instances, blood transfusions can result in additional haemolysis due to immune destruction of transfused RBCs. These haemolytic transfusion reactions which are more likely to occur in CAD can be minimised by transfusing prewarmed blood to 37^0C and starting the transfusion at slower rates.

Warm AIHA often has a chronic and relapsing disease course, therefore, requires early initiation of treatment. The first line of treatment is steroids. In severe haemolysis, the treatment is initiated with intravenous methylprednisolone (0.5-1mg/kg/dose 6-8 hourly for 24-72 hours) or with methylprednisolone pulse therapy (30mg/kg/day for 3 days: a maximum dose of 1g/day). After initial treatment, methylprednisolone is converted to oral prednisolone. Moderate cases can be treated only with oral prednisolone 2mg/kg/day given in 2-3 divided doses. The response to therapy is usually rapid, and approximately 50-80% of patients achieve remission. Once haemoglobin is stabilized at 9-10g/dL, prednisolone can be tailed off by converting to a single daily dose and gradually lowering its dose over 2-4 months. During this period, haematological and biochemical indicators of haemolysis should be carefully monitored. Steroids should be continued until haemoglobin, reticulocyte count and serum haptoglobin are normalized. Many patients tend to relapse if steroids are tailed off too rapidly or discontinued abruptly. DAT can remain weakly positive even when the patient is in disease remission. Persistent positive DAT is suggestive of a secondary cause for AIHA, such as systemic lupus erythematosus or Evans syndrome.

Some patients with warm AIHA have an inadequate response to steroid therapy. In these patients, indications for second-line therapy include not achieving remission after 1-2 months of steroid therapy, relapse during tailing off of steroids, requiring high-dose prednisolone to maintain remission and frequent relapses and remissions that cannot be maintained without prednisolone. Second-line treatment options are rituximab and splenectomy. Rituximab is one of the biological agents, which acts as an anti-CD20 monoclonal antibody and is recommended as the first choice after the failure of steroid therapy. Splenectomy is also effective in controlling the disease and achieving remission in a majority; however, approximately one-third will relapse after 1-2 months following splenectomy. Other treatment options for the refractory disease are intravenous immunoglobulin, danazol, azathioprine, 6-mercaptopurine, cyclosporine, mycophenolate mofetil, tacrolimus, sirolimus, cytotoxic agents like cyclophosphamide and vincristine and several other monoclonal antibodies. However, plasmapheresis is not very effective for warm AIHA.

The mainstay of treatment of CAD is avoiding cold temperature to minimize cold-induced haemolysis. The recommended measures include avoidance of cold rooms, cold drinks, cooling blankets and taking precautions to stay warm during outdoor activities. Underlying infections should be treated with antipyretics and appropriate medications. Severe and symptomatic anaemia requires blood transfusions. Intravenous immunoglobulins and plasmapheresis are other treatment options for severe haemolysis. Rituximab alone or in combination with prednisolone had been used to reduce antibody production.

PCH is a self-limiting disease. Blood transfusions with pre-warmed blood to 37^0C may be required in severe and life-threatening haemolysis. Avoidance of cold environment and cold drinks are also helpful.

Evans syndrome is usually treated with steroids. With prednisolone, 80-85% of patients achieve remission. The second line therapy is similar to refractory warm AIHA.

Follow up and Prognosis

PCH and CAD precipitated by infections are usually self-limiting diseases. In contrast, patients with warm AIHA have a relapsing and chronic disease course. These patients require follow up with close monitoring of haematological and biochemical indicators of haemolysis during tailing off of medication. Monitoring of drug side effects and growth parameters are also important. Factors indicating poor prognosis are family or past history of immune deficiency or autoimmune diseases, concurrent cytopaenias and positive DAT for both IgG and C3d. The mortality rate among children with AIHA is approximately 3-4%. Severe sepsis in splenectomised children, life-threatening bleeding due to severe thrombocytopenia in Evans syndrome and complications of underlying illness are contributing causes for mortality.

Recent Advances

There are new treatment options under investigations. Newer biologics and anti-complement therapy are under research which can be used to treat individuals with refractory cases of AIHA.

REFERENCES

Berentsen, S. 2016. "Cold agglutinin disease." *Hematology Am Soc Hematol Educ Program* 2016 (1):226-231. doi: 10.1182/asheducation-2016.1.226.

Berentsen, S. 2018. "How I manage patients with cold agglutinin disease." *Br J Haematol* 181 (3):320-330. doi: 10.1111/bjh.15109.

Brodsky, R. A. 2019. "Warm Autoimmune Hemolytic Anemia." *N Engl J Med* 381 (7):647-654. doi: 10.1056/NEJMcp1900554.

Go, R. S., J. L. Winters, and N. E. Kay. 2017. "How I treat autoimmune hemolytic anemia." *Blood* 129 (22):2971-2979. doi: 10.1182/blood-2016-11-693689.

Hill, A., and Q. A. Hill. 2018. "Autoimmune hemolytic anemia." *Hematology Am Soc Hematol Educ Program* 2018 (1):382-389. doi: 10.1182/asheducation-2018.1.382.

Kalfa, T. A. 2016. "Warm antibody autoimmune hemolytic anemia." *Hematology Am Soc Hematol Educ Program* 2016 (1):690-697. doi: 10.1182/asheducation-2016.1.690.

Miano, M. 2016. "How I manage Evans Syndrome and AIHA cases in children." *Br J Haematol* 172 (4):524-34. doi: 10.1111/bjh.13866.

Chapter 10

MICROANGIOPATHIC HAEMOLYTIC ANAEMIA

Duantida Songdej*

Ramathibodi Hospital of Mahidol University, Bangkok, Thailand

Microangiopathic haemolytic anaemia (MAHA) is the leading cause of extracorpuscular haemolysis, in which the direct antiglobulin test is negative. MAHA results from a diverse aetiology, however, demonstrates relatively uniform peripheral blood film characteristics irrespective of the cause.

The characteristic features of MAHA in the peripheral blood film is known as MAHA blood picture (Figure 2.5). These features include the presence of burr erythrocytes, schistocytes, helmet cells and microspherocytes which occur in association with varying degree of intravascular haemolysis. There may be associated thrombocytopenia and coagulopathy depending on the aetiology. Laboratory evidence of intravascular haemolysis, such as elevated plasma haemoglobin level,

* Corresponding Author's Email: duantida.son@mahidol.ac.th

absent haptoglobin, haemoglobinuria and increased urine iron excretion is also found. Affected patients may have iron deficiency due to ongoing haemoglobinuria. Treatment should be aimed at improving the underlying cause of MAHA, and red blood cell (RBC) transfusions can be given as needed. Aetiology of MAHA are listed in Table 10.1, and selected causes are described in detail in this chapter.

Table 10.1. Causes of microangiopathic haemolytic anaemia

Group of diseases	Condition
Renal disease	Haemolytic-uremic syndrome Renal vein thrombosis Renal transplantation rejection Radiation nephritis Chronic renal failure
Cardiac conditions	Malignant hypertension Coarctation of aorta Severe valvular heart disease Subacute bacterial endocarditis of aortic valve Intracardiac prosthesis
Liver disease	Severe hepatocellular disease
Infections	Disseminated herpes infection Meningococcal septicaemia Cerebral falciparum malaria
Haematologic disease	Thrombotic thrombocytopenic purpura
Miscellaneous	Severe burns Giant haemangioma (Kasabach-Merritt phenomenon) Disseminated intravascular coagulation of any causes

Kasabach-Merritt Phenomenon

In rare vascular tumours, such as kaposiform haemangioendothelioma and tufted angioma, distorted and rapidly proliferating vascular endothelium results in intralesional haemolytic anaemia along with platelet trapping and activation. Platelet activation subsequently results in the consumption of fibrinogen and other coagulation factors, leading to a high propensity of bleeding. This event is known as the Kasabach-Merritt phenomenon (KMP) and was first described by Kasabach and Merritt in 1940.

Diagnosis

KMP should be considered when there are rapidly enlarging vascular tumours, some of which may be painful. Characteristic laboratory features include low platelet count (commonly ranging between 3-60x10^9/L), low fibrinogen levels, elevated D-dimer and elevated fibrinogen degradation products (FDP). The prothrombin time and activated partial thrombin time (APTT) are typically normal or slightly increased. Anaemia occurs with varying severity due to several causes; haemolytic anaemia secondary to the sheering of RBCs in the abnormal vasculature resulting in MAHA blood picture, intralesional bleeding owing to coagulopathy and sequestration of blood within the tumours.

Treatment

Specific treatment of KMP is targeted at treating the vascular tumour. The supportive treatment includes appropriate consideration of blood component transfusion. Despite profound thrombocytopenia, severe bleeding is rare, and platelet transfusions should be avoided as it can lead to further intralesional platelet trapping and activation. Platelet transfusion should only be given if there is active bleeding or for peri-operative situations. Cryoprecipitate can be given when fibrinogen level is below 1g/L in the presence of active bleeding or for preparation for surgery. Packed RBC transfusion should only be given if anaemia is symptomatic.

Complete surgical resection often is not feasible at the initial stage for most vascular tumours like kaposiform haemangioendothelioma and tufted angioma. This is due to their infiltrative nature and existing coagulopathy due to KMP. Therefore, in most situations, medical treatment is required prior to surgery to decrease the size of tumours and to aim for haemostatic stability in KMP. A variety of regimens have been used to treat kaposiform haemangioendothelioma. These include combinations of steroids, vincristine, aspirin, ticlopidine and interferon-alfa. The decision on which regimen to be used should be extensively discussed between the physicians and the family, based on the availability of the drugs, age of patients, route of administration, potential side effects and cost of the treatment.

Recent Advances

Sirolimus has recently been identified as safe and effective treatment for complicated vascular tumours. It can also be used in children. Previous reports showed that all patients achieve at least partial response in terms of tumour size but with complete and rapid resolution of KMP. Sirolimus is most often used in combination with steroids. Interval blood tests are required to assess sirolimus level and adjust the dose based on the targeted value. Side effects of sirolimus include decreased immunity, mucositis and dyslipidaemia.

Disseminated Intravascular Coagulation

Disseminated intravascular coagulation (DIC) is a condition characterised by evidence of microvascular thrombosis and tendency for bleeding caused by consumptive coagulopathy. Haemolytic anaemia often accompanies this condition as a result of sheering force between RBCs and thrombotic microvasculature of the arterial side. DIC is not isolated but is always secondary to an underlying disease; severe infections and malignancies are the most common aetiologies.

Characteristics of DIC include systemic activation of coagulation resulting in excessive thrombin generation and fibrin deposition. Dysfunction of multiple organ systems is often observed as a consequence of a thrombotic obstruction of small and mid-size vessels. Consumption of platelets, depletion of coagulation factors and imbalance between fibrinolytic and antifibrinolytic systems often lead to severe bleeding. Haemolytic anaemia of varying degree of severity is not uncommon as evidenced by MAHA blood picture in the peripheral blood film. Haemolytic anaemia, however, is not considered in the criteria for the diagnosis of DIC.

Diagnosis

The diagnosis of DIC is based on consensus scoring systems developed by several organizations, including International Society of Thrombosis and Haemostasis, Japanese Society of Thrombosis and Haemostasis, Japanese Ministry of Health, Labour and Welfare and Japanese Association for Acute Medicine. These scoring systems are developed for early detection of DIC and prevention of morbidity and mortality of the condition. Selection of an appropriate scoring system depends on the availability of tests in each institute. In common, scoring systems include platelet number, prothrombin time, fibrinogen and FDP as well as identification of underlying conditions.

Treatment

Correction of the underlying cause is the mainstay of DIC treatment. Transfusion support should be considered for patients with active or high-risk bleeding or for those requiring invasive procedures. In general, the platelet count should be kept above 50×10^9/L in patients with bleeding and $10\text{-}20 \times 10^9$/L in non-bleeding patients. Cryoprecipitate is indicated when fibrinogen is ≤ 1.5g/L, and patients with significant bleeding will benefit from fresh frozen plasma transfusions. RBC transfusions are recommended for symptomatic anaemia. Most importantly, strict monitoring of blood count and coagulation profile (every 6-8 hourly) is recommended in patients with a high risk of bleeding. Unfractionated heparin or low-molecular-weight heparin is recommended for asymptomatic patients as venous thromboembolism prophylaxis but are contraindicated in patients with bleeding. Antifibrinolytic agents are not recommended for asymptomatic patients or patients with organ failure; however, they can be given to patients with hyperfibrinolysis and bleeding.

Recent Advances

New therapeutic agents have recently been introduced to correct pathophysiology of DIC occurring secondary to different underlying causes. These include antithrombin concentrate and recombinant thrombomodulin in sepsis related DIC. However, these agents are not widely available and remain expensive.

Thrombotic Microangiopathy

Thrombotic microangiopathy (TMA) is a group of rare, life-threatening haematological disorders characterised by MAHA, thrombocytopenia and vascular microthrombi formation leading to tissue ischemia. Common forms of TMA are thrombotic thrombocytopenic purpura (TTP) and haemolytic uremic syndrome (HUS). The incidence of TTP in adults is 3 per 1,000,000 population, and the incidence of HUS in children is about 3 per 100,000 population.

Although affected patients with TTP and HUS share characteristic laboratory findings and vascular pathology, aetiology of the two disorders are distinct. TTP results from severe deficiency of enzyme ADAMTS13 (a disintegrin and metalloproteinase with a thrombospondin type 1 motif, member 13) owing to genetic mutations or acquired autoantibodies. The typical form of HUS commonly occurs following diarrhoea caused by Shiga toxin-producing *Escherichia coli* (STEC-HUS). Atypical HUS (aHUS), however, is associated with abnormal host susceptibility to complement-mediated damage.

Diagnosis

Prompt diagnosis of TMA is important, as the condition requires immediate treatment to prevent high morbidity and mortality. MAHA blood picture is the hallmark of TMA and is accompanied by thrombocytopenia. Differences between TTP and HUS diagnostic criteria include organ involvement and specific laboratory investigations to identify the cause (Table 10.2). In clinical practice, however, there is only a small number of patients with full diagnostic criteria. Presence of MAHA blood picture, thrombocytopenia and neurological or renal involvement is sufficient to initiate treatment.

Table 10.2. Diagnostic criteria for thrombotic microangiopathy

	HUS	TTP
Haemoglobin	<10g/dL and haemolysis	
Platelet	Thrombocytopenia	
Organ involvement	Renal failure	Renal failure Neurological symptoms
Specific laboratory investigations	Detection of STEC (STEC-HUS) Genetic abnormality in the complement system (aHUS)	ADAMTS13*<10%

* Test should be performed before initiation of plasma therapy to avoid false-negative results.

Other abnormal laboratory findings involve markers of haemolysis. These are reticulocytosis, elevated lactate dehydrogenase, unconjugated hyperbilirubinemia and low haptoglobin. Direct antiglobulin test is usually negative. Coagulation tests are normal in TMA but may be elevated in patients with very severe symptoms associated with DIC.

TMA and DIC share a number of clinical features in common, leading to misdiagnosis and delayed specific treatment. Table 10.3 compare clinical presentation and laboratory findings of patients with DIC and TMA.

Table 10.3. Comparison of clinical manifestation of DIC and TMA

	DIC	TMA
Clinical presentation		
Organ failure	Often (multiorgan)	Usually (kidney, CNS)
Blood pressure	Low	High
Bleeding tendency	Frequent	Frequent
Haematuria	Sometimes	Frequent
Anaemia	Often	Usually
Laboratory findings		
Platelet count	Low	Low
Haemoglobin	Often low	Low
Prothrombin time	Often prolong	Normal
Fibrin/ FDP	Markedly high	Slightly high
Albumin	Often low	Normal
Lactase dehydrogenase	Often high	High

Treatment

TMA is a medical emergency requiring prompt treatment. Plasmapheresis should be initiated as soon as possible in patients suspected to have TTP. If plasmapheresis is not available, plasma infusion should be administered to replace ADAMTS13 while awaiting transfer to tertiary care. Platelet transfusions should be reserved for those with severe bleeding as it may be associated with increased thrombosis. Prednisolone 1mg/kg/day can be given orally in combination with plasmapheresis if the symptoms, platelet count and haemolytic markers are not improved within 1-2 days. The dose of prednisolone can be tapered off over 3-4 weeks once platelet count reaches normal level. Untreated TTP is associated with a high mortality rate as high as 90% while plasmapheresis reduces it to 20%.

STEC-HUS can be treated with only supportive measures, including fluid rehydration and RBC transfusion. Plasmapheresis is rarely required and is preserved for complicated cases. Antimicrobial therapy may worsen the disease, depending on bacterial strain and antibiotic class. Since the clinical presentation of aHUS is frequently indistinguishable from that of TTP, plasmapheresis should be initially provided for all affected patients.

If a patient does not respond well to plasmapheresis, do not have a very low level of ADAMTS13 and have significant renal impairment, the diagnosis of aHUS is favoured.

Recent Advances

Recent studies in adults show that affected patients with aHUS can be effectively treated with eculizumab, a monoclonal antibody against the terminal complement component C5. Up to 70-80% of patients achieve TMA-free status, and almost 80% can stop dialysis after treatment. Eculizumab is now widely used in children with aHUS, and it yields a comparable outcome to that of adults. There are also recent studies on the use of eculizumab for the treatment of complicated cases of STEC-HUS. Its benefits on STEC-HUS, however, remain controversial and randomized controlled trials are required.

In summary, MAHA can be diagnosed with classical blood pictures and supporting markers of haemolysis. Once the diagnosis is made, it is essential to identify the aetiology of MAHA as this will lead to prompt initial treatment of underlying conditions.

References

Adams, D. M., and K. W. Ricci. 2019. "Vascular Anomalies: Diagnosis of Complicated Anomalies and New Medical Treatment Options." *Hematol Oncol Clin North Am* 33 (3):455-470. doi: 10.1016/j.hoc. 2019.01.011.

Asakura, H., H. Takahashi, T. Uchiyama, Y. Eguchi, K. Okamoto, K. Kawasugi, S. Madoiwa, and H. Wada. 2016. "Proposal for new diagnostic criteria for DIC from the Japanese Society on Thrombosis and Hemostasis." *Thromb J* 14:42. doi: 10.1186/s12959-016-0117-x.

Gando, S., D. Saitoh, H. Ogura, T. Mayumi, K. Koseki, T. Ikeda, H. Ishikura, T. Iba, M. Ueyama, Y. Eguchi, Y. Ohtomo, K. Okamoto, S. Kushimoto, S. Endo, and S. Shimazaki. 2008. "Natural history of disseminated intravascular coagulation diagnosed based on the newly established diagnostic criteria for critically ill patients: results of a multicenter, prospective survey." *Crit Care Med* 36 (1):145-50. doi: 10.1097/01.Ccm.0000295317.97245.2d.

Legendre, C. M., C. Licht, P. Muus, L. A. Greenbaum, S. Babu, C. Bedrosian, C. Bingham, D. J. Cohen, Y. Delmas, K. Douglas, F. Eitner, T. Feldkamp, D. Fouque, R. R. Furman, O. Gaber, M. Herthelius, M. Hourmant, D. Karpman, Y. Lebranchu, C. Mariat, J. Menne, B. Moulin, J. Nürnberger, M. Ogawa, G. Remuzzi, T. Richard, R. Sberro-Soussan, B. Severino, N. S. Sheerin, A. Trivelli, L. B. Zimmerhackl, T. Goodship, and C. Loirat. 2013. "Terminal complement inhibitor eculizumab in atypical hemolytic-uremic syndrome." *N Engl J Med* 368 (23):2169-81. doi: 10.1056/NEJMoa1208981.

Loos, S., J. Oh, and M. J. Kemper. 2018. "Eculizumab in STEC-HUS: need for a proper randomized controlled trial." *Pediatr Nephrol* 33 (8):1277-1281. doi: 10.1007/s00467-018-3972-9.

Mahajan, P., J. Margolin, and I. Iacobas. 2017. "Kasabach-Merritt Phenomenon: Classic Presentation and Management Options." *Clin Med Insights Blood Disord* 10:1179545x17699849. doi: 10.1177/1179545x17699849.

Taylor, F. B., Jr., C. H. Toh, W. K. Hoots, H. Wada, and M. Levi. 2001. "Towards definition, clinical and laboratory criteria, and a scoring system for disseminated intravascular coagulation." *Thromb Haemost* 86 (5):1327-30.

Wada, H., T. Matsumoto, K. Suzuki, H. Imai, N. Katayama, T. Iba, and M. Matsumoto. 2018. "Differences and similarities between disseminated intravascular coagulation and thrombotic microangiopathy." *Thromb J* 16:14. doi: 10.1186/s12959-018-0168-2.

Wada, H., T. Matsumoto, and Y. Yamashita. 2014. "Diagnosis and treatment of disseminated intravascular coagulation (DIC) according to four DIC guidelines." *J Intensive Care* 2 (1):15. doi: 10.1186/2052-0492-2-15.

Wada, H., T. Matsumoto, Y. Yamashita, and T. Hatada. 2014. "Disseminated intravascular coagulation: testing and diagnosis." *Clin Chim Acta* 436:130-4. doi: 10.1016/j.cca.2014.04.020.

Chapter 11

ANAEMIA IN NEONATES

Duantida Songdej*

Ramathibodi Hospital of Mahidol University, Bangkok, Thailand

Anaemia in neonates is diagnosed when the haemoglobin level is lower than minus two standard deviations (-2SD) from the mean for the corresponding gestational and chronological age. Anaemia that occurs during the neonatal period should be considered separately from that happens in older infants and children, due to significant changes happening in red blood cell (RBC) components and physiology from fetal period to the first 3-4 months of life.

From the 12th week of gestation until birth, RBCs compose mainly of haemoglobin (Hb) F ($\alpha_2\gamma_2$). In late gestation, there is an increase in HbA ($\alpha_2\beta_2$) and a gradual decrease in HbF, resulting in 60-80% proportion of HbF and 20-40% of HbA at birth in normal term neonates. HbA_2 ($\alpha_2\delta_2$) is produced from 34-35 weeks of gestation and is found in a small amount at birth. There is an abrupt reduction in the production of haemoglobin and

* Corresponding Author's Email: duantida.son@mahidol.ac.th.

RBCs after birth. This is due to the dramatic decline of erythropoietin levels which occurs as a result of an increase in tissue oxygenation with the first breath of newborns. RBC production rate decreases to its minimum velocity around the second week of life and rises again to the maximum speed at three months of age.

Neonatal RBCs have a shorter lifespan of 60-70 days in comparison to adult RBCs that have a lifespan of 120 days. RBCs of preterm neonates have even shorter lifespans of 35-50 days. Neonatal RBCs are larger in diameter and less deformable compared to adult RBCs. Moreover, blood group surface antigens are expressed less on neonatal RBCs as opposed to adult RBCs.

Table 11.1. Aetiology of neonatal anaemia

Anaemia due to blood loss
Feto-maternal haemorrhage
Twin-to-twin transfusion
Umbilical cord haemorrhages (e.g., Umbilical cord rupture)
Placental haemorrhages (e.g., Placental abruption)
Internal haemorrhage (e.g., Subgaleal haematoma, intracranial haemorrhage)
Anaemia due to red blood cell underproduction
Congenital infection
Nutritional anaemias
Congenital pure red cell aplasia
Haemolytic anaemias
Immune haemolytic anaemia
ABO haemolytic disease of fetus and newborn
Rhesus haemolytic disease of fetus and newborn
Non-immune haemolytic anaemia
Haemoglobin disorders
Membranopathies
Enzymopathies

Table 11.2. Red cell values in the first month of life in the term infant

Age	Haemoglobin (g/dL)		Haematocrit (%)		RBCs ($10^6/\mu L$)		MCV (fL)		MCH (pg)		MCHC (g/dL)		Reticulocyte (%)	
	Mean	-2SD	Mean	-2SD	Mean	-2SD	Mean	-2SD	Mean	-2SD	Mean	-2SD	Mean	-2SD
Birth (cord blood)	16.5	13.5	51	42	4.7	3.9	108	98	34	31	33	30	3.2	1.8
1-3days (capillary)	18.5	14.5	56	45	5.3	4.0	108	95	34	31	33	29	3.0	1.5
1 week	17.5	13.5	54	42	5.1	3.9	107	88	34	28	33	28	0.5	0.1
2 weeks	16.5	12.5	51	39	4.9	3.6	105	86	34	28	33	28	0.5	0.2
1 month	14.0	10.0	43	31	4.2	3.0	104	85	34	28	33	29	0.8	0.4

RBCs; Red blood cells, MCV; Mean corpuscular volume, MCH; Mean corpuscular haemoglobin, MCHC; Mean corpuscular haemoglobin concentration, SD; Standard deviation.

Aetiology

Causes of anaemia in neonates can be subdivided into three main categories; blood loss, underproduction of RBCs and haemolytic anaemias (Table 11.1). Some of these causes are common to infancy and childhood, whereas other conditions, for example, feto-maternal haemorrhage, twin-to-twin transfusion and blood group incompatibilities are found solely in the neonatal period. Instead, other high prevalence causes of anaemia in older children, such as iron deficiency anaemia, are rare in newborns. RBC parameters in the first month of life in the term infant are shown in Table 11.2. Of these, reticulocyte count aids in diagnosing the aetiology, as it is increased in haemolytic anaemia, normal or increased in bleeding and decreased in anaemia due to RBC underproduction.

Anaemia due to Blood Loss

The total blood volume of a healthy term neonates is approximately 80-90mL/kg (body weight). Chronic blood loss, which often occurs prenatally, seldom leads to symptomatic anaemia. In contrast, neonates with acute blood loss of >20% of total blood volume experience unstable vital signs, such as hypotension and tachycardia. Common causes of perinatal blood loss are described below.

Feto-Maternal Haemorrhage

Feto-maternal haemorrhage occurs in minute amounts in 50-75% of normal pregnancies; however, most are clinically insignificant. Neonates with significant chronic feto-maternal blood loss often present with iron deficiency anaemia with hypochromia, microcytosis and anisopoikilocytosis in the peripheral blood film. Low serum ferritin and transferrin saturation are used to confirm the diagnosis.

In contrast, acute feto-maternal haemorrhage often leads to symptomatic anaemia. This condition can be diagnosed by detection of F cells in maternal blood within 24 hours after delivery using the Kleihauer-Betke test (acid elution test). This test can be falsely positive in mothers with thalassaemia or hereditary persistence of fetal haemoglobin.

Twin-to-Twin Transfusion

Twin-to-twin transfusion occurs in 10-15% of monozygotic monochorionic twin pregnancies. The donor twin usually has a bodyweight over 20% lower than the recipient and experience symptomatic anaemia, including heart failure. In contrast, the recipient twin develops polycythaemia and neonatal hyperbilirubinemia at birth. This condition must be considered in the differential diagnosis when twins have >5g/dL difference in their haemoglobin levels.

Umbilical Cord Abnormalities

Umbilical cord abnormalities including umbilical cord rupture in precipitous labour, umbilical cord haematoma, aneurysm, velamentous insertion and vasa previa can lead to neonatal haemorrhage and anaemia.

Placental Abruption

Placental abruption results in bleeding from the fetus and leads to neonatal anaemia.

Internal Haemorrhage

Internal haemorrhages can result from multiple underlying conditions including congenital vascular malformations, congenital bleeding disorders or birth trauma. Locations of bleeding include cephalhaematoma, subgaleal haematoma, intracranial haemorrhage or bleeding into internal organs, such as lungs, liver, spleen and adrenal glands.

Anaemia due to Red Blood Cell Underproduction

Anaemia resulting from the underproduction of RBCs is not very common in the neonatal period. Disease conditions categorised in this group either result in underproduction limited to erythroid lineage or involve white blood cells and platelets as well. The latter is known as bone marrow failure syndromes. Common disorders of RBC underproduction which present in the neonatal period are described below.

Congenital Infection

One-third of primary parvovirus B19 infections in the mother are transmitted to the offspring resulting in fetal anaemia with or without hydrops fetalis or neonatal anaemia.

Nutritional Deficiency

Nutritional deficiency causing anaemia in the newborn period is uncommon. However, iron deficiency can be identified in neonates with chronic blood loss, such as chronic feto-maternal haemorrhage.

Congenital Pure Red Cell Aplasia

Congenital pure red cell aplasia is also known as Diamond-Blackfan anaemia (DBA) or congenital hypoplastic anaemia. The disease is characterised by a block in erythropoiesis at progenitor stage resulting in macrocytic anaemia and reticulocytopenia. Although DBA presents primarily during infancy, 25% of affected cases are found anaemic at birth. Approximately 30-50% of cases are associated with a variety of congenital malformations, including microcephaly, cleft palate, web neck and thumb anomalies. DBA is most frequently (50%) caused by a sporadic mutation in genes encoding ribosomal proteins. The remaining cases are inherited in autosomal dominant pattern with varying phenotypes.

Haemolytic Anaemia

Haemolytic anaemia in the newborn is subdivided into immune or non-immune haemolytic anaemia.

Immune Haemolytic Anaemia

The most common cause of immune haemolytic anaemia is maternal-neonatal blood group incompatibility, which is also known as haemolytic disease of the fetus and newborn (HDFN). HDFN occurs when fetus inherits blood group antigens on RBCs from father that is not compatible with the maternal blood group. Once feto-maternal haemorrhage occurs, maternal antibodies (only IgG type) are produced and form immune complexes on fetal or neonatal RBCs, leading to extravascular haemolysis. The three most common antibodies causing HDFN are anti-D (Rh immunization) and anti-A and anti-B (ABO immunization).

ABO Haemolytic Disease of Fetus and Newborn

Anti-A and anti-B are naturally occurring antibodies; therefore, haemolysis can occur from the first gestation. ABO HDFN occurs only in neonates with blood group A or B, who are born to mothers with blood group O. Haemolysis in this circumstance is less severe than that of Rh HDFN. Affected babies typically present with mild to moderate anaemia and indirect hyperbilirubinemia. This is because there are only small amounts of A and B antigens on neonatal RBCs and anti-A and anti-B are mostly of IgM subtype, which does not cross the placenta. Peripheral blood film typically shows spherocytes and polychromasia. Direct antiglobulin test (DAT) often yield negative or weakly positive results, whereas the indirect antiglobulin test (IAT) often yield positive results.

Rh Haemolytic Disease of Fetus and Newborn

Primary immune response in pregnant women, who are first exposed to D-antigen on fetal RBCs is of IgM antibody subtype. These antibodies do not pass through the placenta; therefore, Rh HDFN is not observed in the first gestation. Later, anti-D IgG is produced in the mother in small amounts which increases rapidly after the second exposure to D-antigen in subsequent gestations. Affected fetuses present with a range of clinical severity, from haemolytic anaemia and indirect hyperbilirubinemia at birth to hydrops fetalis. Peripheral blood film shows numerous nucleated RBCs. This condition is more commonly found in Caucasian.

NON-IMMUNE HAEMOLYTIC ANAEMIA

A vast majority of affected babies in this group have defects in components of RBCs. These include haemoglobin disorders, RBC membrane disorders and RBC enzyme disorders. Affected babies present with a variable degree of anaemia and indirect hyperbilirubinemia at birth. Congenital infections may also lead to non-immune haemolytic anaemia.

Haemoglobin Disorders

The most common haemoglobin disorder that manifests as early as the neonatal period is α-thalassemia. This is because α-globin is the main component of both fetal (HbF) and adult haemoglobin (HbA). Affected individuals with homozygous α^0-thalassaemia (--/--) develop severe anaemia and tissue hypoxia in utero. This often leads to congestive cardiac failure and hydrops fetalis. A vast majority of affected fetuses die in the third trimester of pregnancies or soon after the birth.

Haemoglobin H (HbH) disease is a moderately severe α-thalassemia which is diagnosed when there is only one remaining functional α-globin gene. Affected fetuses survive gestation but present with mild to moderate microcytic anaemia (haemoglobin 11-14 g/dL) at birth. Diagnosis can be made using haemoglobin electrophoresis, which typically shows FABart's pattern with 20-40% of haemoglobin Bart's. Supravital staining may yield negative finding for haemoglobin H inclusion bodies (aggregates of β_4) during the newborn period, as β-globin is expressed at low levels. In rare circumstances, affected fetuses with the non-deletional type of HbH present with hydrops fetalis. Rare cases of homozygous haemoglobin Constant Spring may also present with hydrops fetalis. These affected babies, who were reported to receive intrauterine transfusions, became transfusion-free after the neonatal period. The diagnosis of haemoglobin Constant Spring can be made using genetic analysis.

In contrast, β-thalassemia or sickle cell disease do not present during the neonatal period. Anaemic symptoms typically develop after 6-12 months, when HbF level rapidly decreases.

RBC Membrane Disorders

Hereditary spherocytosis and hereditary elliptocytosis are commonly inherited in the autosomal dominant pattern (~75%). Approximately half of the affected babies experience anaemia and neonatal jaundice. Hepatomegaly and splenomegaly can be observed. Peripheral blood film of these babies and their parents demonstrate specific abnormal RBC shapes, such as spherocytes or elliptocytes.

Affected individuals with hereditary spherocytosis may present with a wide range of clinical severity from mild anaemia to fetal hydrops. Diagnosis can be confirmed using the osmotic fragility test, eosin-5-maleimide (EMA) binding assay performed using flow cytometry or molecular diagnosis of genes encoding RBC membrane proteins. Clinical presentations of hereditary elliptocytosis in childhood and adults are usually mild. EMA binding assay often yields negative results for hereditary elliptocytosis.

Hereditary pyropoikilocytosis is an autosomal recessive form of RBC membrane disorders. Affected individuals inherit homozygous or compound heterozygous mutations of genes encoding RBC membrane proteins, *SPTB* gene being the most common. Clinical presentations include fetal hydrops, severe haemolytic anaemia and jaundice since birth. Most affected individuals became transfusion dependent for life. Peripheral blood film demonstrates anisopoikilocytosis. Elliptocytes are often detected in maternal and paternal blood films. EMA binding assay aids in the diagnosis of affected cases as it mostly yields positive results.

RBC Enzyme Disorders

The most common RBC enzyme disorder is Glucose 6-phosphate dehydrogenase (G6PD) deficiency. Affected individuals are at increased risk of neonatal indirect hyperbilirubinemia. Acute haemolysis after exposure to certain biochemical agents or drugs is less commonly found in the neonatal period. Supravital stain typically shows aggregates of unstable haemoglobin in RBCs, termed Heinz bodies. Diagnosis can be made using the fluorescent spot test or G6PD enzyme assay.

Pyruvate kinase deficiency is an autosomal recessive disorder of RBC enzymes. Approximately 70-80% of affected individuals present with neonatal jaundice which manifest as chronic haemolytic anaemia. Peripheral blood films may be normal or demonstrate echinocytes. Diagnosis can be made using pyruvate kinase enzyme assay.

Infections

Cytomegalovirus, toxoplasmosis, syphilis and bacterial sepsis may trigger haemolytic anaemia in the newborn. Thrombocytopenia is often a co-occurrence in these circumstances. Other clinical features of congenital infections are hepatomegaly, splenomegaly, low birth weight and microcephaly.

Anaemia of Prematurity

In healthy term neonates, haemoglobin level gradually decreases after birth to reach a minimum level of 9.5-11g/dL at 8-12 weeks. This condition is a result of the reduction in erythropoietin level after birth and is referred to as physiologic anaemia of infancy. Physiologic anaemia in preterm infants occurs at 4-8 weeks of age and average haemoglobin level during this period is lower than that of term infants. This is because the mean haemoglobin level of preterm neonates is lower compared to that of term neonates at birth (Table 11.3).

Anaemia of prematurity is caused by multiple factors. Firstly, erythropoietin is produced mainly from the liver during fetal life which is then produced from kidney from the 40th week of gestation. Liver erythropoietin production is less sensitive to hypoxia, resulting in fewer RBC production. Secondly, RBC lifespan in preterm neonates is as short as 35-50 days. Thirdly, the rapid growth of preterm infants requires a large consumption of RBCs. Fourthly, blood drawing for investigations can result in iatrogenic blood loss of significant amounts compared to the total blood volume of preterm babies. Lastly, the preterm neonates have a low level of vitamin E that helps to protect the lipid peroxidation of RBCs.

Anaemia of prematurity can be prevented or relieved by limitation of blood drawing for investigations and vitamin E supplementation. Additionally, delayed umbilical cord clamping has been shown to increase total blood volume in neonates up to 10-15%. Treatment of this condition includes RBC transfusion and erythropoietin injection, together with iron supplementation.

Table 11.3. Red blood cell parameters in preterm neonates of different gestational ages

Week of gestation	Haemoglobin (g/dL)	RBCs ($X10^6/\mu L$)	Haematocrit (%)	MCV (fL)
18-21	11.7 ± 1.3	2.9 ± 0.4	37.3 ± 4.3	131.1 ± 11
22-25	12.2 ± 1.6	3.1 ± 0.3	38.6 ± 3.9	125.1 ±7.8
26-29	12.9 ± 1.4	3.5 ± 0.4	40.9 ± 4.4	118.5 ± 8.0
>30	13.6 ± 2.2	3.8 ± 0.6	43.6 ± 7.2	114.4 ± 9.3

Treatment of Anaemia in Neonates

The mainstay of treatment of anaemia in neonates is to correct the cause of anaemia. Indication for RBC transfusion depends on different factors. These include the velocity of blood loss (acute vs chronic), symptoms related to tissue hypoxia such as tachycardia, metabolic acidosis and poor weight gain, apnoea and requirement of oxygen support or mechanical ventilation.

There are many guidelines for blood transfusion in terms infants; British Committee for Standards in Haematology (2016), American Red Cross (2007), Australian National Blood Authority (2016), Canadian Blood Services (2017) and Dutch Guidelines Quality Council (2019). In clinical practice, these guidelines can be adapted to suit each hospital setting. An example of the transfusion threshold from British Committee for Standards in Haematology (2016) is shown in Table 11.4.

Table 11.4. Suggested transfusion threshold for term neonates from British Committee for Standards in Haematology (BCSH, 2016)

Postnatal week	On respiratory support	No respiratory support
Week 1	<10-12 g/dL	<10 g/dL
Week 2	<9.5-10 g/dL	<7.5 g/dL
Week ≥3	<8.5-10g/dL	<7.5 g/dL

The blood product used in neonates should be leukocyte-depleted RBCs to prevent febrile non-haemolytic transfusion reactions, human leukocyte antigen (HLA) alloimmunization and CMV infection. Indications for the use of irradiated blood products are intrauterine transfusion, postnatal exchange transfusion or top-up transfusion following intrauterine transfusion, blood products from first- or second-degree relatives and transfusion for neonates suspected of having immunodeficiency. These irradiated blood products prevent transfusion-associated graft-versus-host disease.

Table 11.5. Suggested transfusion threshold for preterm neonates <32 weeks of gestation by British Committee for Standards in Haematology (2016)

Postnatal age	Suggested transfusion threshold (haemoglobin- g/dL)		
	Ventilated	On oxygen/ NIPPV	Off oxygen
First 24 h	<12	<12	<10
Day 1-7	<12	<10	<10
Day 8-14	<10	<9.5	<7.5*
Day 15 onward	<10	<8.5	<7.5*

NIPPV: non-invasive positive pressure ventilation.

* Clinician may use up to 8.5 g/dL depending on clinical situation.

Recent Advances

From 2016, BCSH recommended a new transfusion trend for preterm neonates with gestational age <32 weeks, which is known as 'restrictive transfusion' (Table 11.5). Restrictive transfusion results in a reduction of RBC products used without adverse effect on mortality and morbidity rates of the preterm.

REFERENCES

Aher, S., K. Malwatkar, and S. Kadam. 2008. "Neonatal anemia." *Semin Fetal Neonatal Med* 13 (4):239-47. doi: 10.1016/j.siny.2008.02.009.

Bizzarro, M. J., E. Colson, and R. A. Ehrenkranz. 2004. "Differential diagnosis and management of anemia in the newborn." *Pediatr Clin North Am* 51 (4):1087-107, xi. doi: 10.1016/j.pcl.2004.03.006.

Brugnara, C. and O. S. Platt (2009). "The neonatal erythroyte and its disorders." In: Orkin, S. H., D. G., Nathan, D. Ginsberg, A. T., Look, D. E., Fisher, S. E., Lux, eds. *Nathan and Oski's Hematology of Infancy and Childhood.* 7th ed. Philadelphia: Saunders Elsevier; 21-66.

Gibson, B. E., A. Todd, I. Roberts, D. Pamphilon, C. Rodeck, P. Bolton-Maggs, G. Burbin, J. Duguid, F. Boulton, H. Cohen, N. Smith, D. B. McClelland, M. Rowley, and G. Turner. 2004. "Transfusion guidelines for neonates and older children." *Br J Haematol* 124 (4):433-53. doi: 10.1111/j.1365-2141.2004.04815.x.

He, Y., Y. Zhao, J. W. Lou, Y. H. Liu, and D. Z. Li. 2016. "Fetal Anemia and Hydrops Fetalis Associated with Homozygous Hb Constant Spring (HBA2: c.427T>C)." *Hemoglobin* 40 (2):97-101. doi: 10.3109/03630269.2015.1126721.

Howarth, C., J. Banerjee, and N. Aladangady. 2018. "Red Blood Cell Transfusion in Preterm Infants: Current Evidence and Controversies." *Neonatology* 114 (1):7-16. doi: 10.1159/000486584.

Lorey, F., P. Charoenkwan, H. E. Witkowska, J. Lafferty, M. Patterson, B. Eng, J. S. Waye, J. Z. Finklestein, and D. H. Chui. 2001. "Hb H hydrops foetalis syndrome: a case report and review of literature." *Br J Haematol* 115 (1):72-8. doi: 10.1046/j.1365-2141.2001.03080.x.

Maheshwari, A., R. M. Patel, and R. D. Christensen. 2018. "Anemia, red blood cell transfusions, and necrotizing enterocolitis." *Semin Pediatr Surg* 27 (1):47-51. doi: 10.1053/j.sempedsurg.2017.11.009.

Strauss, R. G. 2008. "How I transfuse red blood cells and platelets to infants with the anemia and thrombocytopenia of prematurity." *Transfusion* 48 (2):209-17. doi: 10.1111/j.1537-2995.2007.01592.x.

Chapter 12

OTHER NORMOCYTIC ANAEMIAS

Sachith Mettananda* and Tharindi Suriapperuma
Department of Paediatrics, University of Kelaniya, Ragama, Sri Lanka

PHYSIOLOGICAL ANAEMIA OF INFANCY

Physiological anaemia, as the name implies is a non-pathological condition causing anaemia in normal term infants. The highest haemoglobin concentration (14.5-22.5g/dL) at any age of a normal human is observed soon after birth. From the first week of life, haemoglobin concentration gradually drops to reach a nadir of 9-10g/dL around 6-12 weeks, which is referred to as physiological anaemia of infancy.

The primary pathophysiological mechanism of physiological anaemia is the suppression of erythropoiesis due to increased delivery of oxygen to tissues. With the first breath, the arterial oxygen saturation rises from 50% to above 95% in normal healthy neonates. Similarly, a physiological switch of haemoglobin from fetal haemoglobin (HbF) to adult haemoglobin

---

* Corresponding Author's Email: sachith.mettananda@kln.ac.lk.

(HbA) occurs during the first few months of life. In comparison to HbF, HbA has a lower affinity to oxygen, thus facilitating oxygen delivery to tissues. The resultant improvement in tissue oxygenation leads to downregulation of erythropoietin and suppression of erythropoiesis resulting in physiological anaemia. The haemoglobin drops until tissue oxygen demand exceeds the oxygen delivery at which point the erythropoietin production increases and the erythropoiesis resumes.

The usual presentation of physiological anaemia is incidental detection of low haemoglobin in an otherwise healthy asymptomatic infant with no or mild pallor. Except for low haemoglobin, red blood cell (RBC) indices and other cell lines are normal. Features that would suggest a pathological process in an infant presenting with anaemia during this age are; symptoms of anaemia, signs of haemolysis, organomegaly, haemoglobin less than 9g/dL and abnormalities in RBC indices or other cell lines. Patients with physiological anaemia should be reassured, and no medical intervention is indicated. Haemoglobin level will gradually rise to normal (above 11.0g/dL) by six months.

Transient Erythroblastopenia of Childhood

Transient erythroblastopenia of childhood (TEC) is the most prevalent acquired red blood cell aplasia in children which is particularly common between 6 months to 4 years. Most patients are above the age of 12 months; however, only 10% present after three years. The reported annual incidence is 4.3 cases per 100,000 with a male to female ratio of 1.2: 1.

Aetiology

TEC is characterized by a temporary cession of erythropoiesis leading to a transient RBC aplasia which is usually self-limiting. The exact aetiology of this is unclear; however, is believed to be an interplay between genetic factors, environmental triggers and immune mechanisms. The role of genetic predisposition in the pathogenesis of TEC is evident by reports of familial cases and co-occurrence in identical twins. Several viruses including parvovirus B19, human herpesvirus type 6 and echovirus 11 have been reported to be associated with TEC.

Clinical Manifestations

TEC results in gradual onset anaemia which is moderate to severe. Most patients are asymptomatic but can have clinically detectable pallor. There are no other abnormal physical signs; a feature that is important in differentiating this from congenital pure red cell aplasia. However, patients with severe anaemia due to TEC can develop fatigability, tachycardia and flow murmur.

Investigations

Investigations will show low haemoglobin in the range of 5-7g/dL with normal MCV and marked reticulocytopenia. The neutrophil count is usually normal, but mild neutropoenia is reported in some children with TEC. Platelet count is normal or elevated. Peripheral blood film shows normocytic normochromic anaemia with normal erythrocyte morphology. Direct Coombs test is negative. Bone marrow aspiration biopsy is rarely indicated nonetheless, if performed, shows reduction or absence of erythrocyte precursors. The laboratory features that would differentiate TEC from Diamond Blackfan anaemia are normal MCV, HbF percentage and erythrocyte adenosine deaminase activity and the lack of RBC i antigen.

Treatment

Almost all individuals with TEC recover spontaneously without sequelae in 1-2 months, a fact that also confirms its diagnosis. Severely affected symptomatic children will require blood transfusion occasionally but needing more than one blood transfusion is extremely rare and indicative of alternative diagnoses. Corticosteroids have no place in the treatment of TEC.

CONGENITAL DYSERYTHROPOIETIC ANAEMIA

Congenital dyserythropoietic anaemia (CDA) is a rare group of inherited anaemias that demonstrate heterogeneous clinical presentation. These anaemias are characterised by ineffective erythropoiesis, multinuclear erythroblasts, haemolysis and secondary hemochromatosis. Three main types of CDA which are differentiated based on the morphological abnormalities of RBC and erythroblasts and genetic mutations are described. Although CDA is classified under normocytic anaemia in this text, some types of CDA produce macrocytic anaemias.

Congenital Dyserythropoietic Anaemia I

CDA I is an autosomal recessive disorder caused by homozygous or compound heterozygous mutations in the *CDAN1* gene. It usually presents during the first decade of life with clinical features of moderate pallor, jaundice, splenomegaly and hepatomegaly. Skeletal deformities are present in one-third of patients while cholelithiasis and secondary haemosiderosis develop later in life. Inappropriate suppression of hepcidin increases iron absorption by intestinal enterocytes which exacerbates target organ damage due to iron overload.

Full blood count of patients with CDA I confirms anaemia and high MCV (100-120fL); however, some children have normocytic RBC indices. Blood film shows macrocytes, elliptocytes and anisopoikilocytosis. The reticulocyte count is inadequate for the degree of anaemia, and serum haptoglobin is low. Bone marrow aspiration reveals erythroid hyperplasia, megaloblastosis and bi- or multi-nucleated polychromatic erythroblasts with inter-nuclear chromatin bridges in incompletely divided cells. Electron microscopy studies of bone marrow show 'swiss cheese' or spongy appearance of heterochromatin and invaginations of cytoplasm into the nucleus.

Treatment of CDA I is primarily supportive. Approximately half of the patients will require blood transfusions and 3-4% are transfusion dependent. Interferon-α is effective in reducing the transfusion requirement in some patients. Splenectomy is generally not indicated nor beneficial. Allogeneic haematopoietic stem cell (HSC) transplantations from human leukocyte antigen (HLA)-identical siblings have been successful in a few cases.

Congenital Dyserythropoietic Anaemia II

CDA II is the most common CDA type. This autosomal recessive disease is caused by homozygous or compound heterozygous mutations in the *SEC23B* gene. Clinical features of CDA II are similar to that of CDA I; however, the diagnosis is usually made later in life because the symptoms are milder. Severely affected patients may present during fetal life with hydrops fetalis.

Full blood counts of patients with CDA II show mild anaemia, normal to increased MCV and inappropriately low reticulocytosis. Anisopoikilocytosis, basophilic stippling and binucleated erythroblasts are seen in the peripheral blood film. Binucleated cells are present in the bone marrow with hypercellularity and erythroid hyperplasia. Compared to CDA I, bone marrow contains 10-35% of binucleate erythroblasts with few multinucleated forms. The pathognomonic feature is lysis of patient RBCs in acidified serum due to IgM antibody that recognizes an antigen present on CDA II cells but not on normal cells. Due to the technical difficulties of this test, the diagnosis is made by analysing RBC membrane proteins by sodium dodecyl sulphate-polyacrylamide gel electrophoresis (SDS-PAGE). Approximately, 10% of patients with CDA II require blood transfusions.

Other treatment options are splenectomy and allogeneic HSC transplantation; both have reported favourable results.

Congenital Dyserythropoietic Anaemia III

CDA III is the least common variant. It is due to autosomal dominantly inherited or de novo mutations of the *KIF23* gene. CDA III is characterised by intravascular haemolysis; therefore, it is not associated with splenomegaly or clinically significant iron overload. Blood film will have macrocytic RBCs, whereas bone marrow shows erythroid hyperplasia with giant erythroblasts containing multiple (up to 12) nuclei. Blood transfusions are generally not required for CDA III.

Paroxysmal Nocturnal Haemoglobinuria

Paroxysmal nocturnal haemoglobinuria (PNH) is an acquired disorder of HSCs which is mostly reported among adults and rarely in children. Males and females are equally affected. Somatic mutations of the *PIGA* gene that encodes for glycosyltransferase in HSCs are responsible for PNH. Glycosyltransferase is essential in the biosynthesis of glycosylphosphatidylinositol, an anchoring protein which attaches specific proteins to the cell surface. Absence or near absence of glycosylphosphatidylinositol and glycosylphosphatidylinositol-anchored proteins CD59 and CD55 that protect erythroid cells from complement-mediated haemolysis is the primary pathophysiological mechanism of PNH. Deficiency of CD59 leads to complement-mediated intravascular haemolysis, whereas the reduction in CD55 results in complement-mediated extravascular haemolysis by reticuloendothelial macrophages in the liver and spleen.

Clinical Manifestations

The cardinal clinical manifestations of PNH are haemolysis, thrombosis and bone marrow failure. Haemolysis in PNH is characteristically intravascular which occur in paroxysms at night leading to haemoglobinuria manifesting as nocturnal dark urine. However, a majority of children with PNH have chronic haemolysis throughout the day. Common clinical features related to haemolysis are fatigue, dyspnoea, icterus and dark red or cola-coloured urine. Additionally, patients with PNH display clinical features related to smooth muscle dystonia, for example, abdominal pain, dysphagia and erectile dysfunction, due to the depletion of nitric oxide attributed to scavenging effects of free haemoglobin.

Thrombosis is the leading cause of mortality in patients with PNH. Venous thrombosis is commoner than arterial thrombosis and occurs in intra-abdominal sites such as hepatic, portal, splenic and mesenteric veins and inferior vena cava as well as in cerebral sinuses and dermal veins. The most common site of thrombosis is hepatic vein causing Budd-Chiari syndrome while deep vein thrombosis and pulmonary embolism are also not uncommon.

Bone marrow failure and impaired haematopoiesis causing pancytopenia is a frequent feature of PNH. Pulmonary hypertension due to nitric oxide depletion and pulmonary emboli, acute kidney injury and chronic kidney disease due to nephrotoxic effects of haem and aseptic meningitis and arthralgia due to immune mechanisms are other features of PNH. PNH is not a malignant disease, but a sub-set of patients with PNH develop acute leukaemia, most commonly acute myeloid leukaemia.

Investigations

Haematological and biochemical investigations in patients with PNH show evidence of intravascular haemolysis; low haemoglobin, reticulocytosis, indirect hyperbilirubinaemia and elevated lactate dehydrogenase. Haptoglobin level is low and free haemoglobin is evident in the serum and urine. Direct Coombs test is negative. Bone marrow aspiration biopsy is not essential for the diagnosis; however, it is required in patients with pancytopenia. It characteristically shows hypocellular bone marrow but, normocellular and hypercellular marrow with erythroid hyperplasia can be seen in some patients. Demonstration of reduced levels of glycosylphosphatidylinositol-anchored proteins on erythrocytes and polymorphonuclear cells in peripheral blood samples using flowcytometry confirms the diagnosis of PNH.

Classification

PNH is divided into three types based on the clinical presentation;

- 'Classic PNH' which is characterized by intravascular haemolysis and thrombotic episodes without other bone marrow abnormalities
- 'PNH in the setting of another bone marrow failure syndrome' shows evidence of haemolysis with another bone marrow abnormality such as aplastic anaemia or myelodysplastic syndrome
- 'Subclinical PNH' is characterised by a small population of haematopoietic cells lacking glycosylphosphatidylinositol-anchored proteins but without clinical or laboratory evidence of haemolysis

Treatment

Treatment of PNH is primarily using anti-complement therapy. Eculizumab, a humanized monoclonal antibody which binds to the complement component C5 and inhibits the formation of membrane attack complex has shown to reduce intravascular haemolysis, need for blood transfusions and risk for thrombosis while improving quality of life in patients with PNH. It is considered in patients with disabling fatigue, thrombosis, transfusion dependence, frequent symptoms of smooth muscle dystonia and renal insufficiency. Ravulizumab is another monoclonal antibody that can be used as anti-complement therapy.

Patients with severe anaemia with cardiovascular compromise may require a blood transfusion. Iron supplementation should be given for patients who are iron deficient and routine folic acid supplementation is recommended to the patients with chronic haemolysis. Acute thrombosis is managed with heparin or low-molecular-weight heparin in addition to eculizumab. Individuals who have life-threatening complications such as severe aplastic anaemia, myelodysplastic syndromes, and complications unresponsive to anti-complement therapy are candidates for HSC transplantation.

ANAEMIA OF CHRONIC DISEASE

Anaemia of chronic disease is caused by a number of chronic disorders with ongoing inflammation such as chronic infections, autoimmune disorders and malignancies. The primary pathophysiology is reduced availability of iron for erythropoiesis which is mediated by elevated hepcidin and high level of cytokines released by the persistent inflammatory response. Hepcidin prevents absorption of iron by enterocytes and release of iron from reticuloendothelial cells. Additionally, high levels of cytokines suppress bone marrow and inhibit erythropoiesis and promote the destruction of RBCs by macrophage engulfment. Moreover, interleukin-1 promotes macrophages to engulf RBCs and destroy them.

Investigations

Anaemia of chronic disease results in mild to moderate anaemia with normocytic and normochromic RBCs. Serum iron profile shows low serum iron and total iron-binding capacity with normal to low transferrin saturation. Serum ferritin, as well as c-reactive protein and erythrocyte sedimentation rate, are elevated due to ongoing inflammation. The absolute reticulocyte count is normal or low. Soluble transferrin receptors are normal in anaemia of chronic disease helping to differentiate it from iron deficiency. Anaemia of chronic disease is a hyperproliferative anaemia with normocellular bone marrow with reduced erythrocyte precursors.

Treatment

The mainstay of treatment is to treat the underlying condition when possible. Blood transfusions are rarely required but can be used to improve haemoglobin temporarily. Iron supplementation is indicated to patients with iron deficiency. Recombinant erythropoiesis-stimulating agents such as erythropoietin have doubtful benefits.

Anaemia of Renal Disease

Anaemia is an inevitable complication of chronic kidney disease. It develops when the glomerular filtration rate drops below 30-50mL/min per $1.73m^2$. Decreased erythropoietin production by renal erythropoietin producing cells is the primary cause for anaemia of renal disease. Additionally, iron deficiency due to inadequate nutritional intake, reduced intestinal absorption attributed to upregulation of hepcidin and chronic blood loss from frequent phlebotomies and haemodialysis contribute to anaemia. Also, erythropoietin dysregulation, other associated nutritional deficiencies such as vitamin B12, folate, carnitine and vitamin C and haemolysis induced by uraemia and oxidative stress are important pathophysiological mechanisms of anaemia of renal disease.

Investigations

Annual screening for anaemia should be performed in all children with chronic kidney disease. Children with anaemia of renal disease have normocytic RBC indices and normal to low absolute reticulocyte count. Ferritin will be low in the presence of iron deficiency and high if there is associated inflammation.

Treatment

Erythrocyte-stimulating agents and iron supplementation are the current options to treat anaemia of renal disease. Therapy should be aimed at maintaining haemoglobin at 11-12g/dL. Erythrocyte-stimulating agents include recombinant human erythropoietin and darbepoetin alfa, a long-acting synthetic form of erythropoietin. Recombinant human erythropoietin is administered subcutaneously (initial dose 20-50IU/kg) 1-3 times per week while darbepoetin alfa can be given weekly or bi-weekly. Iron supplementation can be given orally or parenterally. Oral iron supplementation is efficacious in most of the children with chronic kidney disease; however, children with more advance disease who require haemodialysis benefit from intravenous preparations of iron.

References

Atkinson, M. A., and B. A. Warady. 2018. "Anemia in chronic kidney disease." *Pediatr Nephrol* 33 (2):227-238. doi: 10.1007/s00467-017-3663-y.

Brodsky, R. A. 2014. "Paroxysmal nocturnal hemoglobinuria." *Blood* 124 (18):2804-11. doi: 10.1182/blood-2014-02-522128.

Gambale, A., A. Iolascon, I. Andolfo, and R. Russo. 2016. "Diagnosis and management of congenital dyserythropoietic anemias." *Expert Rev Hematol* 9 (3):283-96. doi: 10.1586/17474086.2016.1131608.

Hill, A., A. E. DeZern, T. Kinoshita, and R. A. Brodsky. 2017. "Paroxysmal nocturnal haemoglobinuria." *Nat Rev Dis Primers* 3: 17028. doi: 10.1038/nrdp.2017.28.

Iolascon, A., H. Heimpel, A. Wahlin, and H. Tamary. 2013. "Congenital dyserythropoietic anemias: molecular insights and diagnostic approach." *Blood* 122 (13):2162-6. doi: 10.1182/blood-2013-05-468223.

Iolascon, A., R. Russo, and J. Delaunay. 2011. "Congenital dyserythropoietic anemias." *Curr Opin Hematol* 18 (3):146-51. doi: 10.1097/MOH.0b013e32834521b0.

Moreno-Carralero, M. I., S. Horta-Herrera, M. Morado-Arias, M. P. Ricard-Andrés, A. Lemes-Castellano, M. Abio-Calvete, M. T. Cedena-Romero, F. A. González-Fernández, L. Llorente-González, A. M. Periago-Peralta, S. de-la-Iglesia-Íñigo, M. Méndez, and M. J. Morán-Jiménez. 2018. "Clinical and genetic features of congenital dyserythropoietic anemia (CDA)." *Eur J Haematol* 101 (3):368-378. doi: 10.1111/ejh.13112.

Parker, C. J. 2016. "Update on the diagnosis and management of paroxysmal nocturnal hemoglobinuria." *Hematology Am Soc Hematol Educ Program* 2016 (1):208-216. doi: 10.1182/asheducation-2016.1.208.

Roy, N. B. A., and C. Babbs. 2019. "The pathogenesis, diagnosis and management of congenital dyserythropoietic anaemia type I." *Br J Haematol* 185 (3):436-449. doi: 10.1111/bjh.15817.

Part 4.
Macrocytic Anaemias

Chapter 13

MEGALOBLASTIC ANAEMIA

Sachith Mettananda*[*] and Tharindi Suriapperuma
Department of Paediatrics, University of Kelaniya, Ragama, Sri Lanka

Megaloblastic anaemia is a form of macrocytic anaemia characterised by megaloblastic erythropoiesis due to impaired metabolism of nucleic acids. Slowing of nuclear maturation and division cycles relative to the cytoplasm of erythroid precursor cells results in cells with large and immature nuclei. The deficiency of nutrients, inborn errors of metabolism and medications that interfere with purine and pyrimidine metabolism cause megaloblastic anaemia; however, the two most common causes are deficiencies of vitamin B12 and folate.

METABOLISM OF VITAMIN B12 AND FOLATE

Vitamin B12 (cobalamin) and folate are water-soluble vitamins which cannot be synthesized in human cells. However, a normal balanced diet

[*] Corresponding Author's Email: sachith.mettananda@kln.ac.lk.

contains adequate amounts of these vitamins to fulfil the recommended daily intake, which is 2.4μg for vitamin B12 and 400μg for folate in adults. Vitamin B12 is present exclusively in animal products; meats, dairy products, eggs and liver are rich sources of vitamin B12. Conversely, dark green leafy vegetables and many plants and animal products contain folate.

Vitamin B12 bound to proteins in food is released in the stomach due to the acidic nature of the gastric fluid. Liberated vitamin B12 is then bound to haptocorrin, which is secreted in saliva. In the upper small intestine, pancreatic proteases cleave off haptocorrin to release vitamin B12 which in turn is bound to intrinsic factor produced by the gastric parietal cells. This vitamin B12 and intrinsic factor complex are absorbed by the mucosal receptors in the ileum. Absorbed vitamin B12 is released into the circulation where it is bound by transcobalamin to be transported to tissues. This complex is taken up into cells and is converted to adenosylcobalamin or methylcobalamin intracellularly.

Body vitamin B12 levels drop in the first few months after birth to reach the lowest level around 4-6 months of age. After six months, the vitamin B12 level increases again to reach a peak between 3-7 years. Thereafter, during adolescence, vitamin B12 levels start to drop again. Body stores of vitamin B12 are approximately 2-5mg, of which half is stored in the liver. The stores are adequate for nearly two years.

Folate in food is in the form of folate polyglutamate which are cleaved to folate monoglutamates before being absorbed in the jejunum. Once absorbed, folate is reduced to dihydrofolate and tetrahydrofolate to be effective in its physiological functions. The total body store of folate is approximately 0.5-20mg, which is adequate only for weeks to a few months.

AETIOLOGY

Vitamin B12 and folate deficiency are the most common causes of megaloblastic anaemia in children. The deficiency of vitamin B12 could be due to several reasons. Firstly, the inadequate intake of vitamin B12 causes vitamin B12 deficiency. Individuals who are on strict vegetarian diets are at high risk of developing vitamin B12 deficiency. Next, conditions that result in impaired secretion of gastric acid or pepsin, for example, gastrectomy or bariatric surgery lead to vitamin B12 deficiency. Due to a lack of gastric acid and pepsin, the liberation of vitamin B12 from food protein is impaired. Pernicious anaemia is another common cause of vitamin B12 deficiency. It is an autoimmune disorder due to anti-intrinsic factor or anti-parietal cell antibodies. Additionally, some medications like proton pump inhibitors, H_2 receptor blockers and antacids reduce the gastric acid secretion, thus decreasing the availability of vitamin B12. Pancreatic enzymes are required to dissociate vitamin B12 from salivary or food proteins and allow vitamin B12 to bind with intrinsic factor. Chronic pancreatic insufficiency may impair the above process.

Small intestinal surgery and inflammation can restrict the surface of absorption of vitamin B12. Small intestinal bacterial overgrowth, inflammatory bowel disease, radiation enteritis, coeliac disease, tuberculous ileitis, lymphoma involving the small intestine and ileal resection due to various reasons can give rise to a restriction of the absorptive surface resulting in vitamin B12 deficiency. Infestation with fish tapeworm causes vitamin B12 deficiency by competing with vitamin B12 absorption. Finally, Imerslund-Gräsbeck syndrome (juvenile megaloblastic anaemia) is a rare genetic cause for vitamin B12 deficiency in children.

With regards to folate, inadequate dietary intake is a well-recognized cause of folate deficiency in children. Restrictive diet, anorexia nervosa and chronic alcohol use are some of the predisposing factors. Malabsorption due to various malabsorption syndromes, for example, coeliac disease and tropical sprue lead to folate deficiency. Limited absorptive surface following intestinal resection is also a recognized cause of folate deficiency. Medications that interfere with folate metabolism, for example, methotrexate, antibiotics such as trimethoprim and pyrimethamine and some antiseizure medications are well-known causes of folate deficiency. Increased requirement of folate in conditions with rapid cell proliferation such as chronic haemolytic anaemia, exfoliative skin diseases, pregnancy, lactation and haemodialysis can cause folate deficiency as they have increased demand of folate for DNA synthesis. Finally, rare genetic disorders that interfere with folate absorption and metabolism are also identified.

Pathophysiology

During erythropoiesis, differentiating erythroid precursors undergo rapid cell divisions and become progressively smaller as they mature. This process demands accelerated DNA synthesis; therefore, conditions that lead to impaired synthesis of DNA, for example, vitamin B12 and folate deficiency result in a delay in nuclear maturation compared to the cytoplasm. This asynchrony leads to the formation of large, immature nuclei relative to the cytoplasm with megaloblastic changes in erythroid precursors. Myeloid and platelet precursors are also affected giving rise to giant metamyelocytes, leukopenia and thrombocytopenia.

Clinical Manifestations

The main clinical features of megaloblastic anaemia are similar irrespective of the cause. Typical patients present with symptoms of anaemia which depends on the severity and the rate of development. Most patients have nonspecific symptoms such as fatigability, irritability and changes in cognition. If the anaemia is severe, features of tissue hypoxia such as shortness of breath and chest pain appear. A mild degree of haemolysis causing jaundice combined with pallor will give rise to the lemon-yellow colour of the body.

Neurological manifestations are commonly associated with vitamin B12 deficiency; however, neurocognitive manifestations can also occur in folate deficiency. Vitamin B12 deficiency results in demyelination of peripheral and central neurons leading to symmetrical paraesthesia or numbness of limbs and abnormal gait. Subacute combined degeneration of the dorsal and lateral columns of the spinal cord is a classic association confined to vitamin B12 deficiency. The symptoms of the above condition are progressive weakness, ataxia and paraesthesia, which can progress into spasticity and paraplegia. There could be many associated neuropsychiatric manifestations such as mood changes, depression, irritability, cognitive impairment and psychosis. Visual disturbances, impaired sensation of vibration and proprioception and extrapyramidal signs (e.g., dystonia, dysarthria, rigidity) are also reported with vitamin B12 deficiency. In some children with neuropsychiatric manifestations, red cell morphology can be normal without evidence of anaemia. Thus, the absence of haematological abnormalities does not exclude vitamin B12 deficiency. Other rare features associated with vitamin B12 deficiency are skin pigmentation, osteoporosis and fractures.

Infants with vitamin B12 deficiency may present with feeding difficulties, regurgitation, constipation, apathy, irritability and developmental delay. Older children can present with weight loss, impaired mental and social development and poor school performance. Symptoms related to the gastrointestinal tract are due to inability to provide the required demand of vitamins for rapid cell turnover. Vitamin B12 deficiency can cause glossitis, and folate deficiency may result in oral ulcers.

Neonates with deficiency of vitamin B12 or folate may present with developmental delay or regression, abnormal tone, specially hypotonia, feeding difficulties, tremors and sometimes convulsions. There are known consequences due to low maternal vitamin B12 in the newborn such as developmental delay, cerebral atrophy and hypotonia. They are more prone to get cardiovascular diseases, neurodegenerative disorders and psychiatric illnesses as adults possibly due to increased levels of homocysteine.

Investigations and Diagnosis

Megaloblastic anaemia is suspected in a child with unexplained anaemia which is associated with macrocytic RBC morphology, strict vegetarian diet, neurological or psychiatric symptoms or other autoimmune disorders. Full blood count features of megaloblastic anaemia are low haemoglobin and increased MCV along with mild leukopenia and thrombocytopenia. MCV >115fL is highly suggestive megaloblastic anaemia due to vitamin B12 or folate deficiency. However, a normal MCV does not exclude vitamin B12 or folate deficiency. Peripheral blood film shows macrocytic red blood cells (RBCs) with oval macrocytes and hyper segmented neutrophils. Megaloblastic anaemia also leads to premature destruction of erythrocytes within the bone marrow and in circulation. Therefore, biochemical features of haemolysis such as indirect hyperbilirubinaemia, low haptoglobin and elevated lactate dehydrogenase may be evident. However, unlike in other haemolytic anaemias, reticulocyte count is low or normal in megaloblastic anaemia.

Serum vitamin B12 and folate levels are required to differentiate vitamin B12 deficiency from folate deficiency. Serum B12 level above 300pg/mL is normal while a level below 200pg/mL confirms the diagnosis of vitamin B12 deficiency; a level between 200 to 300pg/mL is borderline. Serum folate level above 4ng/mL is normal; 2-4 ng/mL is borderline, and a value below 2ng/mL is consistent with folate deficiency. RBC folate level, which reflects the folate status of erythrocytes over its lifetime is a better indicator of folate status than serum folate level as it is not affected by dietary changes.

Additional tests are done only in selected individuals. Methylmalonyl-CoA is converted to succinyl-CoA in the presence of vitamin B12 by methylmalonyl-CoA mutase. In vitamin B12 deficiency, methylmalonic acid (MMA) level is elevated. In the presence of both vitamin B12 and folate, homocysteine is converted to methionine. Consequently, elevated homocysteine levels are seen in both vitamin B12 and folate deficiencies. Therefore, the elevation of both MMA and homocysteine suggest vitamin B12 deficiency, whereas the elevation of only homocysteine is associated with folate deficiency. However, several other conditions cause elevation of MMA, for example, renal insufficiency and methylmalonic acidaemia.

If the tests are borderline and the clinical suspicion is high, treatment trial of the suspected vitamin deficiency is recommended. Depending on the response to vitamin replacement, retrospective diagnosis can be made. The haematological response is demonstrated by a rise in haemoglobin and a high reticulocyte count two weeks after treatment.

Once the diagnosis of either vitamin B12 deficiency or folate deficiency is made, further investigations are indicated to identify the underlying aetiologies such as coeliac disease, inflammatory bowel disease and pancreatic insufficiency. Antibodies against intrinsic factor can be measured to diagnose pernicious anaemia. Schilling test, which was done in the past to diagnose pernicious anaemia is no longer recommended. Bone marrow examination is generally not required to diagnose vitamin B12 or folate deficiency.

Differential Diagnosis

The differential diagnosis of megaloblastic anaemia includes other causes of macrocytic anaemia, pancytopenia or hypersegmented neutrophils and conditions presenting with anaemia and neuropsychiatric manifestations. Other causes of macrocytosis are presented in chapter 14 and 15. Bone marrow hypoplasia syndromes and autoimmune disorders can present with nonspecific symptoms similar to vitamin B12 or folate deficiency. Bone marrow examination is required if these disorders are suspected. Conditions that have co-occurrence of neuropsychiatric manifestations and haematological abnormalities include copper deficiency, systemic lupus erythematosus, hypothyroidism and hepatic encephalopathy. However, these conditions could easily be differentiated from megaloblastic anaemia by other clinical manifestations.

Treatment

Most children with vitamin B12 and folate deficiency are asymptomatic and identified incidentally; therefore, the deficiencies can be corrected over weeks. However, children with symptomatic anaemia, neurologic or neuropsychiatric manifestations and those who present during neonatal period or infancy require prompt treatment. Very rare instances of severe anaemia with haemodynamic instability should be urgently treated with blood transfusions.

Treatment of vitamin B12 deficiency in children is with therapeutic doses of vitamin B12, which can be administered intramuscularly or deep subcutaneously. Vitamin B12 is available as cyanocobalamin or hydroxocobalamin in therapeutic preparations. It is recommended to administer 50-100μg of parenteral vitamin B12 once a week until the deficiency is corrected. Thereafter treatment is continued either as cyanocobalamin once a month or hydroxocobalamin once every two months. The duration of treatment depends on the aetiology of vitamin B12 deficiency. Lifelong treatment is indicated in children with irreversible conditions such as pernicious anaemia, ileal resection and gastric bypass surgery. However, if the aetiology is reversed, vitamin B12 treatment can be stopped once the deficiency is corrected.

Folate deficiency in children is treated with oral folic acid 1-5mg daily. If the cause of folate deficiency is reversible, the treatment is continued for 1-4 months or until laboratory evidence of haematological recovery. However, if the folate deficiency is due to a chronic illness, treatment is given lifelong. Intravenous preparation of folic acid is available for rapid and urgent correction of folate in symptomatic patients but is not widely used in children.

Response to vitamin B12 or folate therapy is rapid with evidence of reticulocytosis in 3-4 days, rise in haemoglobin in 1-2 weeks, the disappearance of hypersegmented neutrophils in 2 weeks, resolution of leukopenia and thrombocytopenia in 2-4 weeks and normalisation of haemoglobin in 4-8 weeks. Emotional lability and irritability of vitamin B12 deficiency improve rapidly; however, neurological deficits will take a longer duration to respond. In most instances, paraesthesia without sensory loss and motor weakness will recover completely.

The reduced form of folate is known as folinic acid (leucovorin). It is used to prevent drug toxicity, especially following methotrexate and should not be used in the treatment of folate deficiency. Another important point that should be noted is that folic acid treatment could partially correct the hematologic abnormalities and mask the presence of vitamin B12 deficiency. As folic acid is not effective in reversing neurologic manifestations of vitamin B12 deficiency, delay in treatment can worsen the neurologic complications. Therefore, it is recommended to exclude vitamin B12 deficiency in children with folate deficiency before the commencement of therapy.

PREVENTION

Deficiencies of vitamin B12 and folate could easily be prevented by supplementation of the at-risk population. Oral vitamin B12 supplementation is recommended to children who are on strict vegetarian diets, those who have undergone gastric surgery and to neonates born to mothers with vitamin B12 deficiency. Folic acid supplementation is given to children with malabsorption, chronic gastrointestinal disorders and conditions resulting in high cell turnover, for example, chronic haemolytic anaemia and atopic eczema. Oral folic acid 1mg daily is sufficient to prevent folate deficiency in these individuals.

FOLLOW UP

Individuals with pernicious anaemia are prone to develop other autoimmune disorders, autoimmune thyroid disease in particular, therefore, should frequently be screened for these. Some patients who had severe neurological manifestations before treatment could have permanent neurological sequelae. These complications need to be monitored during follow up.

References

Gräsbeck, Ralph. 2006. "Imerslund-Gräsbeck syndrome (selective vitamin B12 malabsorption with proteinuria)." *Orphanet Journal of Rare Diseases* 1 (1):17. doi: 10.1186/1750-1172-1-17.

Green, R. 2017. "Vitamin B (12) deficiency from the perspective of a practicing hematologist." *Blood* 129 (19):2603-2611. doi: 10.1182/blood-2016-10-569186.

Green, R., L. H. Allen, A. L. Bjørke-Monsen, A. Brito, J. L. Guéant, J. W. Miller, A. M. Molloy, E. Nexo, S. Stabler, B. H. Toh, P. M. Ueland, and C. Yajnik. 2017. "Vitamin B (12) deficiency." *Nat Rev Dis Primers* 3:17040. doi: 10.1038/nrdp.2017.40.

Sobczyńska-Malefora, Agata, and Dominic J Harrington. 2018. "Laboratory assessment of folate (vitamin B₉) status." *Journal of Clinical Pathology* 71 (11):949-956. doi: 10.1136/jclinpath-2018-205048.

Stabler, Sally P. 2013. "Vitamin B12 Deficiency." *New England Journal of Medicine* 368 (2):149-160. doi: 10.1056/NEJMcp1113996.

Venkatramanan, S., I. E. Armata, B. J. Strupp, and J. L. Finkelstein. 2016. "Vitamin B-12 and Cognition in Children." *Adv Nutr* 7 (5):879-88. doi: 10.3945/an.115.012021.

Chapter 14

RED BLOOD CELL APLASIA

Duantida Songdej*

Ramathibodi Hospital of Mahidol University, Bangkok, Thailand

Red blood cell (RBC) aplasia is a condition characterised by anaemia due to defects in proliferation and development of bone marrow haematopoietic stem cells (HSCs) or erythroid precursor cells. Affected patients usually present with normochromic and normocytic or macrocytic anaemia and reticulocytopenia. RBC aplasia can be divided into two main groups depending on the number of cell lineage involved;

1. Pure RBC aplasia
2. RBC aplasia with other cell lineages involvement

* Corresponding Author's Email: duantida.son@mahidol.ac.th.

Pure Red Blood Cell Aplasia

Haematological abnormalities of pure RBC aplasia are confined to the RBC lineage. Causes of pure RBC aplasia are summarised in Table 14.1.

Table 14.1. Aetiology of pure red blood cell aplasia

Aetiological category	Syndrome or disease condition
Congenital	Diamond Blackfan anaemia Congenital dyserythropoietic anaemia (see Chapter 12) Pearson syndrome
Acquired	
Idiopathic	Transient erythroblastopenia of childhood (see Chapter 12)
Secondary	Parvovirus B19 infection Drugs or toxins Malnutrition Thymoma Collagen vascular disorders/ autoimmune associated Malignant associated

Red Blood Cell Aplasia with Other Cell Lineages Involvement

A number of disorders are involved in the defective production of not only erythroid cells, but also myeloid or megakaryocytic cells. A failure of all three cell lines resulting in pancytopenia with hypoplastic or aplastic bone marrow is the principal manifestation of these disorders. Aetiology of RBC aplasia with other cell lineages involvement is summarised in Table 14.2.

Table 14.2. Aetiology of RBC aplasia with other cell lineages involvement

Aetiological category	Syndrome or disease condition
Congenital	Fanconi anaemia Dyskeratosis congenita Shwachman Diamond syndrome (predominantly neutropenia)
Acquired Idiopathic Secondary	 Drugs Predictable, dose-dependent and reversible: 6-Mercaptopurine, methotrexate, cyclophosphamide, busulfan, chloramphenicol Unpredictable and in normal doses: Chloramphenicol, sulphonamides, mephenytoin, hydantoin, phenylbutazone, gold, tolbutamide, chlorpropamide, quinacrine Chemicals Benzene, carbon tetrachloride, glue, toluene Insecticides DDT, parathion, chlordane Toxins Radiation Infections Viral hepatitis, HIV, epstein-barr virus, rubella, measles, mumps, cytomegalovirus (newborn), herpes virus (newborn), chronic parvovirus Immunologic disorders Graft versus host reaction in transfused immunologically incompetent subjects, X-linked lymphoproliferative syndrome, eosinophilic fasciitis, hypogammaglobulinemia Aplastic anaemia preceding acute leukaemia Myelodysplastic syndromes Malnutrition Pregnancy

Diamond Blackfan Anaemia

Genetics and Pathophysiology

Diamond Blackfan anaemia (DBA) results from autosomal dominant pathogenic variants in genes encoding small)40S(or large)60S(ribosomal subunits leading to haploinsufficiency of ribosomal proteins. Consequent defects in ribosome biosynthesis lead to the death of erythroid progenitors and precursors by apoptosis. So far, with the help of next-generation sequencing, at least 18 genes encoding for ribosomal proteins are identified. These include, but may not be limited to *RPS19, RPS24, RPS7, RPS15, RPS27A, RPS10, RPS29* and *RPS26* that encode for proteins in the small ribosomal subunit, and *RPL5, RPL11, RPL35A, RPL15* and *RPL26* encoding for proteins in the large ribosomal subunit. Among these genes, *RPS19* is the most common genetic cause of DBA, accounting for 25% of the cases. More recently, pathogenic variants in the *GATA1* gene on the X-chromosome has also been identified as a cause of DBA in a minority of patients.

Clinical Manifestations

A vast majority of the patients present with severe macrocytic anaemia during the first year of life with a median age of presentation of 2 months. A small number of affected infants may be anaemic at birth. Most patients have normal platelet and white blood cell counts. Associated congenital abnormalities are found in approximately half of the patients with short stature and craniofacial malformation being the most common accounting for 50%. Other abnormalities include upper limb and hand deformities, cardiac malformations and urogenital defects. However, the severity of clinical presentation can vary widely, and asymptomatic carriers of pathogenic variants in DBA-associated genes have been reported. DBA is also associated with increased risk of cancer, including myelodysplastic syndrome (MDS), acute myeloid leukaemia (AML), osteosarcoma, colon cancer and female genital cancers. These patients can also develop aplastic anaemia.

Diagnosis

DBA is often suspected by the presentation of infantile or early childhood-onset severe and persistent macrocytic anaemia with reticulocytopenia. Elevated erythrocyte adenosine deaminase activity (eADA) is found in approximately 85% of the patients. Elevated fetal haemoglobin (HbF) is often detected and is useful for identification of potential asymptomatic carriers, especially in family members of affected individuals. Bone marrow biopsy typically reveals normocellularity or slight hypocellularity with the absence of normoblasts. Lymphoid, granulocytic and megakaryocytic lineages are usually normal.

Treatment

Oral corticosteroid has been reported to induce remission in up to 80% of the patients with DBA. Prednisolone 2mg/kg/day in single or divided doses is used to initiate treatment. When haemoglobin level reaches 10g/dL, the dose should be reduced to a minimum dose necessary to maintain a reasonable haemoglobin level. Steroid-related side effects should be closely monitored, as these patients usually require treatment for long periods. Corticosteroids should be avoided in the first year of life. These younger patients are given packed RBC transfusions as the primary treatment.

RBC transfusion should be given as required. Leukocyte-depleted packed RBC should be used to reduce the incidence of non-haemolytic febrile transfusion reactions as well as human leukocyte antigen (HLA) alloimmunization. Effective iron chelation is typically recommended after 10-15 transfusions. The oral iron chelator deferiprone has been reported to cause neutropenia in DBA; therefore, should be avoided. End organ damage resulting from iron overload should be optimally monitored.

HLA-matched related or unrelated-donor haematopoietic stem cell (HSC) transplantation should be considered for patients with DBA who are refractory to steroid therapy or transfusion-dependent and for those who developed leukaemia, MDS or aplastic anaemia. A family bone marrow donor must be screened for DBA-associated mutations to rule out asymptomatic carrier status.

Prognosis

Spontaneous remission of DBA has been reported in up to 25% of the patients by the age of 25 years independent of the pattern of response to treatment. The overall survival at the age of 40 years is 75.1±4.8%. Death in DBA is most often due to treatment-related complications, such as end-organ damage caused by iron overload and infection related complications of HSC transplantation.

Recent Advances

As impaired DNA translation due to ribosomal insufficiency is considered as a defect in DBA, amino acid L-leucine, a translation enhancer, has been investigated as a potential therapy. The recent clinical data has demonstrated an increase in the haemoglobin level and transfusion independence in patients with DBA following L-leucine therapeutic use. A phase I/II clinical trial of L-leucine in DBA patients has been completed, and a phase II study is ongoing (ClinicalTrials.gov identifier NCT02386267).

Parvovirus B19-Associated Pure Red Cell Aplasia

Parvovirus B19 directly binds to the human RBC surface P antigen and infects erythroid progenitors. The virus can cause an aplastic crisis in patients with chronic haemolytic disorders, such as sickle cell anaemia, thalassaemia and hereditary spherocytosis. Moreover, the virus can cause chronic pure red cell aplasia in immunocompromised patients.

Fanconi Anaemia

Genetics and Pathophysiology

Fanconi anaemia is the most frequent inherited aplastic anaemia which is caused by germline mutations in DNA repair genes of the FA/BRCA pathway leading to chromosomal instability. This results in haematopoietic failure, birth defects and cancer predisposition in affected patients. Currently, pathogenic variants in at least 20 key DNA repair genes have been identified; *FANCA* being the most common followed by *FANCC* accounting for 65% and 14% patients with Fanconi anaemia respectively. Fanconi anaemia-associated genes are inherited in an autosomal recessive pattern, except for *FANCB* which is inherited in an X-linked recessive mode. The heterozygote carrier frequency of Fanconi anaemia is estimated to be 1 in 300 in the general population. All racial and ethnic groups are affected.

Clinical Manifestations

Patients with Fanconi anaemia often have short stature and skin abnormalities that include café-au-lait patches, hyperpigmentation and hypopigmented spots. Approximately two-thirds of patients have congenital anomalies including thumb abnormalities, absent or hypoplastic radius, microcephaly, triangular face, renal and heart anomalies and VACTERL-H association (Vertebral anomalies, anal atresia, cardiac defects, tracheo-oesophageal fistula, oesophageal atresia, renal abnormalities, limb abnormalities and hydrocephalus).

Variable degree of pancytopenia usually develops in childhood with a median age of presentation of 8-10 years. Approximately 40% of the patients with Fanconi anaemia develop severe bone marrow failure by the age of 20 years. Haematologic manifestations include macrocytosis followed by thrombocytopenia often leading to progressive pancytopenia and severe aplastic anaemia. The main features in bone marrow examination are hypocellularity and fatty replacement. Additionally, dysplastic erythroid and myeloid precursors, as well as abnormal megakaryocytes, can be found in residual haematopoiesis.

Patients with Fanconi anaemia have nearly 800-fold increase in the relative risk of developing AML or MDS and a higher risk of developing non-haematologic cancers at a younger age, when compared to general population. These non-haematologic cancers include squamous cell carcinoma of the head and neck and malignancies in the breast, kidney, lung, colon, bone, eyes and female gynaecological organs.

Diagnosis

Laboratory evaluation for Fanconi anaemia should be performed in all children with aplastic anaemia, MDS or AML, in patients with classical congenital anomalies associated with Fanconi anaemia, in patients who develop Fanconi anaemia-associated cancers at a younger age and in siblings of patients with Fanconi anaemia. Screening test includes the identification of increased chromosomal breakage in peripheral blood T-lymphocytes cultured in the presence of DNA cross-linking agents such as mitomycin C or diepoxybutane. Recent advance in next-generation sequencing, array comparative genomic hybridization and multiplex ligation-dependent probe amplification allow identification of pathogenic mutations in Fanconi anaemia-associated genes leading to a definite diagnosis.

Treatment

Androgen (oxymetholone 2-5mg/kg/day) has been reported to improved blood count and reduce the requirement of blood transfusions in

60-70% of the patients. Therefore, androgen is often used for Fanconi anaemia-associated bone marrow failure in patients awaiting HSC transplantation or in patients who cannot undergo HSC transplantation.

Packed RBCs and platelet transfusions should be minimized and reserved for patients who do not respond to androgen therapy. Blood products should be irradiated and leukocyte-depleted when possible. Iron status should be monitored regularly, and iron chelation should be given for chronically transfused patients.

As patients with Fanconi anaemia have a higher chance of development of MDS and AML, interval surveillance with bone marrow aspiration and biopsy is recommended. The aims are to look for dysplastic changes of the bone marrow cell morphology, presence of blast cells and abnormal cytogenetics.

HSC transplantation is a primary therapeutic option for bone marrow failure in patients with Fanconi anaemia. The optimal timing for HSC transplantation is prior to progressive cytopenia and the occurrence of clonal evolution. Potential HSC donors in family members should be genetically screened for Fanconi anaemia prior to transplantation. The patients and their family members should also be counselled that HSC transplantation is associated with post-transplant solid malignancies and morbidity associated with graft-versus-host disease. Patients with Fanconi anaemia who develop MDS or AML require standard-dose chemotherapy followed by reduced-intensity conditioning regimen HSC transplantation. The outcome of HSC transplantation in this group of patients is poor.

Recent Advances

Targeted gene therapy and cell reprogramming in Fanconi anaemia is under experimental trials.

Dyskeratosis Congenita

Genetics and Pathophysiology

Patients with dyskeratosis congenita have pathogenic mutations in the genes which are involved in telomere biology, resulting in deficient telomerase activity leading to short telomeres. Telomerase activity is found in tissues with rapid turnover rates such as the basal layer of the epidermis, squamous epithelium of oral cavity, type 2 alveolar epithelium and haematopoietic progenitors. As a result, defects or premature cancer in these tissues are observed in patients with dyskeratosis congenita.

DKC1 is the most common gene in which pathogenic variants that are inherited in X-linked recessive pattern are found. The second most common gene is *TINF2,* of which the mutations are inherited in an autosomal dominant pattern. A minority of pathogenic variants causing dyskeratosis congenita are inherited as autosomal recessive mutations.

Clinical Manifestations

Dyskeratosis congenita has a wide variability of clinical presentations. However, the diagnosis of classical dyskeratosis congenita is often made in the presence of a clinical triad; reticular skin pigmentation, nail dysplasia and oral leucoplakia. Other clinical manifestations include bone marrow failure, pulmonary fibrosis, oesophageal and urethral stenosis, liver disease, premature grey hair and avascular necrosis of the hip.

Bone marrow failure occurs in 86% of the patients with dyskeratosis congenita and is the cause of death in a majority. The median age at onset of pancytopenia is approximately ten years. The anaemia is associated with macrocytosis and elevated fetal haemoglobin. A significant number of patients who do not die of bone marrow failure die as a result of pulmonary fibrosis with or without HSC transplantation.

Up to 9% of the patients develop MDS, AML or Hodgkin disease. The most common solid cancer is squamous cell carcinoma of head and neck, followed by anorectal, stomach and lung cancers. Neurological symptoms such as cerebellar hypoplasia, microcephaly, developmental delay and central nervous system calcification can be found in some severe forms of dyskeratosis congenita, known as Hoyeraal-Hreidarsson (HH) and Revesz syndromes (RS).

Diagnosis

Dyskeratosis congenita is diagnosed clinically in the presence of at least two of the mucocutaneous triad, or one classic triad plus one of the other dyskeratosis congenita-associated features. However, clinical manifestations of dyskeratosis congenita may occur over time and may not be present at the same time. Therefore, laboratory diagnosis is beneficial. The presence of leucocyte telomere length less than the first percentile for the age, when measured by flow cytometry with fluorescence in situ hybridization (flow FISH), can be used as laboratory criteria for diagnosis.

Treatment

Supportive measures include transfusion of blood products as required similar to those given to other bone marrow failure syndromes. Oral androgen therapy (oxymetholone) has been used for the management of cytopenias in dyskeratosis congenita with variable responses. Surveillance bone marrow aspiration and cytogenetic studies are recommended annually in patients with dyskeratosis congenita for monitoring of MDS or AML. An HLA-matched related or an alternative donor HSC transplantation should be considered in those patients with progression of cytopenias or development of MDS or AML. The reduced intensity or non-myeloablative conditioning regimens should be used to decrease chemotherapy-related side effects. However, patients with dyskeratosis congenita are at higher risk of developing pulmonary complication following HSC transplantation as compared to patients with other diseases. The median survival of patients with dyskeratosis congenita is approximately 40-50 years.

Recent Advances

Gene therapy, which aims to correct short telomeres in inherited bone marrow failure syndromes remains in the pre-clinical phase.

ACQUIRED IDIOPATHIC APLASTIC ANAEMIA

Epidemiology

Aplastic anaemia is characterized by hypocellular bone marrow and peripheral cytopenia, which is either inherited or acquired. The incidence of acquired aplastic anaemia is two per million in Western countries and 4-6 per million in Asia. Among acquired aplastic anaemias, 70% are idiopathic in nature. However, a number of aetiologies causing acquired aplastic anaemia such as drugs, toxin, viral infections and radiation should be ruled out prior to the diagnosis of idiopathic aplastic anaemia (Table 14.2). In this section, aplastic anaemia refers to acquired idiopathic aplastic anaemia.

Genetics and Pathophysiology

Many clinical and laboratory studies suggest that aplastic anaemia results from immune-mediated destruction of haematopoietic progenitors. T lymphocytes play a central role by secreting γ-interferon and tumour necrosis factor, both of which exert direct toxicity to haematopoietic progenitors, interrupt their mitotic cycle and lead progenitors to undergo an apoptotic process. Although acquired idiopathic aplastic anaemia is not overtly genetic, it is likely that affected patients have a genetic predisposition to bone marrow failure.

Clinical Manifestations

Clinical symptoms and signs are related to pancytopenia. These include fatigue and pallor owing to anaemia, presence of petechiae, bruises and mucocutaneous bleeding due to thrombocytopenia and susceptibility to infection and oral mucositis owing to neutropenia. Liver and spleen are normal. Leukaemia must be ruled out in the presence of hepatosplenomegaly.

Diagnosis

Aplastic anaemia is diagnosed and categorised as non-severe, severe and very severe using peripheral blood and bone marrow core biopsy criteria as shown in Table 14.3.

Table 14.3. Criteria for diagnosis of acquired aplastic anaemia

Severity	Criteria
Non-severe	Peripheral blood: 2 of 3 values WBC ≤3,500/μL and ANC ≤1,500/μL Platelet ≤50,000/μL Anaemia with corrected reticulocytes < 1% Hypocellular marrow not met severe aplastic anaemia criteria
Severe	Peripheral blood : 2 of 3 values ANC ≤ 500/μL Platelet ≤ 20,000/μL Anaemia with corrected reticulocytes < 1% Marrow cellularity ≤ 25%
Very severe	The same as severe aplastic anaemia except for ANC < 200/μL

Fetal haemoglobin may be slightly to moderately elevated. Megaloblastic changes of erythroid precursors from bone marrow examination are often seen. Importantly, inherited bone marrow failure syndromes and primary diseases that cause aplastic marrow must be investigated and excluded prior to the diagnosis of idiopathic aplastic anaemia. These investigations include, but not limited to, thorough physical examination to look for inherited bone marrow failure-associated congenital abnormalities, chromosomal breakage assay, telomere length study and viral serology testing for hepatitis A, B and C, epstein-barr virus, parvovirus B19, cytomegalovirus and HIV.

Treatment

Patients with severe and very severe aplastic anaemia should be upfront treated with allogeneic HSC transplantation if HLA-matched related donor is available. In the absence of such donor, immunosuppressive therapy composing of anti-thymocyte globulin, cyclosporine A and methylprednisolone to prevent serum sickness should be given as soon as possible. Granulocyte colony-stimulating factor is sometimes used to achieve a more rapid increment in granulocyte count. Haematologic responses to the immunosuppressive therapy are typically assessed at three months after treatment. If there is no response and the patients remain transfusion-dependent, a search for an alternative donor for HSC transplantation should be performed. Alternatively, a second course of immunosuppressive therapy can be given with a lower chance of response as compared to that given in the first course. Patients receiving immunosuppressive therapy should also receive *Pneumocystis jeroveci* prophylaxis with trimethoprim and sulfamethoxazole.

Patients with non-severe aplastic anaemia should be observed with close follow-up and must be given supportive care. Androgen therapy (oxymetholone) and prednisolone have been used for these patients with variable responses. Once these patients develop severe aplastic anaemia along with severe thrombocytopenia causing significant bleeding, chronic anaemia requiring regular transfusions and serious infections, treatment similar to severe aplastic anaemia should be initiated.

Also, supportive treatment in patients with aplastic anaemia is crucial. These include transfusion of packed RBC and platelet products as required and comprehensive monitoring and treatment of infections. Organisms that cause severe infections in affected patients can be bacteria, virus and fungus.

Recent Advances

Recent studies have shown that eltrombopag, a synthetic thrombopoietin-receptor agonist can result in significant improvement in blood count in affect patients with aplastic anaemia, who are refractory to immunosuppressive therapy alone. At present, there are on-going large clinical trials testing combination therapy of anti-thymocyte globulin, cyclosporine A and eltrombopag in both adults and children, who are newly diagnosed with aplastic anaemia or refractory to the first course of immunosuppressive therapy.

References

Alter, B. P., G. M. Baerlocher, S. A. Savage, S. J. Chanock, B. B. Weksler, J. P. Willner, J. A. Peters, N. Giri, and P. M. Lansdorp. 2007. "Very short telomere length by flow fluorescence in situ hybridization identifies patients with dyskeratosis congenita." *Blood* 110 (5):1439-47. doi: 10.1182/blood-2007-02-075598.

Ballew, B. J., and S. A. Savage. 2013. "Updates on the biology and management of dyskeratosis congenita and related telomere biology disorders." *Expert Rev Hematol* 6 (3):327-37. doi: 10.1586/ehm.13.23.

Gambale, A., A. Iolascon, I. Andolfo, and R. Russo. 2016. "Diagnosis and management of congenital dyserythropoietic anemias." *Expert Rev Hematol* 9 (3):283-96. doi: 10.1586/17474086.2016.1131608.

Kallen, M. E., A. Dulau-Florea, W. Wang, and K. R. Calvo. 2019. "Acquired and germline predisposition to bone marrow failure: Diagnostic features and clinical implications." *Semin Hematol* 56 (1):69-82. doi: 10.1053/j.seminhematol.2018.05.016.

Khincha, P. P., I. M. Wentzensen, N. Giri, B. P. Alter, and S. A. Savage. 2014. "Response to androgen therapy in patients with dyskeratosis congenita." *Br J Haematol* 165 (3):349-57. doi: 10.1111/bjh.12748.

Means, R. T., Jr. 2016. "Pure red cell aplasia." *Blood* 128 (21):2504-2509. doi: 10.1182/blood-2016-05-717140.

Paustian, L., M. M. Chao, H. Hanenberg, D. Schindler, H. Neitzel, C. P. Kratz, and W. Ebell. 2016. "Androgen therapy in Fanconi anemia: A retrospective analysis of 30 years in Germany." *Pediatr Hematol Oncol* 33 (1):5-12. doi: 10.3109/08880018.2015.1129567.

Sankaran, V. G., R. Ghazvinian, R. Do, P. Thiru, J. A. Vergilio, A. H. Beggs, C. A. Sieff, S. H. Orkin, D. G. Nathan, E. S. Lander, and H. T. Gazda. 2012. "Exome sequencing identifies GATA1 mutations resulting in Diamond-Blackfan anemia." *J Clin Invest* 122 (7):2439-43. doi: 10.1172/jci63597.

Savage, S. A., and C. Dufour. 2017. "Classical inherited bone marrow failure syndromes with high risk for myelodysplastic syndrome and acute myelogenous leukemia." *Semin Hematol* 54 (2):105-114. doi: 10.1053/j.seminhematol.2017.04.004.

Townsley, D. M., P. Scheinberg, T. Winkler, R. Desmond, B. Dumitriu, O. Rios, B. Weinstein, J. Valdez, J. Lotter, X. Feng, M. Desierto, H. Leuva, M. Bevans, C. Wu, A. Larochelle, K. R. Calvo, C. E. Dunbar, and N. S. Young. 2017. "Eltrombopag Added to Standard Immunosuppression for Aplastic Anemia." *N Engl J Med* 376 (16):1540-1550. doi: 10.1056/NEJMoa1613878.

Wegman-Ostrosky, T., and S. A. Savage. 2017. "The genomics of inherited bone marrow failure: from mechanism to the clinic." *Br J Haematol* 177 (4):526-542. doi: 10.1111/bjh.14535.

Young, N. S., R. T. Calado, and P. Scheinberg. 2006. "Current concepts in the pathophysiology and treatment of aplastic anemia." *Blood* 108 (8):2509-19. doi: 10.1182/blood-2006-03-010777.

Chapter 15

OTHER MACROCYTIC ANAEMIAS

Sachith Mettananda*

Department of Paediatrics, University of Kelaniya, Ragama, Sri Lanka

Macrocytosis and macrocytic anaemia results from three main mechanisms. Firstly, impaired DNA synthesis and nuclear development due to deficiencies in folate or vitamin B12 result in megaloblastic anaemia (described in chapter 13). Secondly premature release of reticulocytes into the circulation cause increase in MCV due to relatively large cell volume of these cells. Thirdly, abnormalities of the molecular constituents of the erythroid membrane, lipid abnormalities, in particular, lead to increased cell volume and macrocytosis. In this chapter, we will briefly describe the rare causes of macrocytic anaemia in children.

* Corresponding Author's Email: sachith.mettananda@kln.ac.lk

Hypothyroidism

The mechanism of macrocytosis in hypothyroidism is unclear, however, it is believed to be an interplay between bone marrow depression, decreased erythropoietin production and concomitant vitamin B_{12} or folate deficiency. Anaemia is mild and, in some patients, macrocytosis is observed without anaemia.

Down Syndrome

Patients with trisomy 21 have macrocytic cells, although accompanying anaemia is generally not present.

Liver Diseases

Liver disease causes macrocytosis and macrocytic anaemia by effects on the lipid composition of the RBC membrane. In addition to macrocytic anaemia, patients with liver disease commonly have thrombocytopenia.

Myelodysplastic Syndrome

Myelodysplastic syndrome (MDS) is a rare group of disorders in children with an annual incidence of 1-4 cases per million. It is a clonal hematopoietic disorder characterized by peripheral cytopenia, ineffective haematopoiesis and an increased risk of progression to acute myeloid leukaemia. Childhood MDS is often associated with inherited bone marrow failure syndromes or genetic predisposition syndromes. Pancytopenia with a severe decrease of bone marrow cellularity is the hallmark of this disorder. In contrast to adults who usually present with isolated anaemia, hematologic manifestations in children frequently include thrombocytopenia and neutropenia. In addition, the MCV is elevated, and haemoglobin F levels are elevated. Allogeneic HSC transplantation is a curative treatment for many patients with MDS and should be considered as the treatment of choice if there is an indication for therapy, and a suitable donor is identified.

REFERENCES

Cascio, M. J., and T. G. DeLoughery. 2017. "Anemia: Evaluation and Diagnostic Tests." *Med Clin North Am* 101 (2):263-284. doi: 10. 1016/j.mcna.2016.09.003.

Kivivuori, S. M., J. Rajantie, and M. A. Siimes. 1996. "Peripheral blood cell counts in infants with Down's syndrome." *Clin Genet* 49 (1):15-9. doi: 10.1111/j.1399-0004.1996.tb04318.x.

Moore, C. A., and A. Adil. 2020. "Macrocytic Anemia." In *StatPearls*. Treasure Island (FL): StatPearls Publishing Copyright © 2020, StatPearls Publishing LLC.

Szczepanek-Parulska, E., A. Hernik, and M. Ruchała. 2017. "Anemia in thyroid diseases." *Pol Arch Intern Med* 127 (5):352-360. doi: 10. 20452/pamw.3985.

Part 5.
Polycythaemia

Chapter 16

CHILDHOOD POLYCYTHAEMIA

Tharindi Suriapperuma and Sachith Mettananda *

Department of Paediatrics, University of Kelaniya, Ragama, Sri Lanka

Polycythaemia refers to an abnormal elevation in haemoglobin, haematocrit, red blood cell (RBC) count and total RBC volume in the peripheral blood. It is defined as an elevation of RBC mass >25% above the mean normal value based on body surface area or a haemoglobin level >16.5g/dL in adult men or >16g/dL in adult women.

AETIOLOGY AND CLASSIFICATION

Polycythaemia could be relative or absolute. Relative polycythaemia refers to an increase in the haematocrit or haemoglobin due to a decrease in the plasma volume. It occurs as a result of haemoconcentration, most

* Corresponding Author's Email: sachith.mettananda@kln.ac.lk.

commonly due to acute dehydration, burns, plasma leakage and diuretic use.

Absolute polycythaemia is characterised by elevated RBC mass due to increased RBC production. Causes of absolute polycythaemia can be categorised into two groups; primary polycythaemia and secondary polycythaemia (Table 16.1). Primary polycythaemia is caused by genetic mutations of erythroid progenitor cells that result in hypersensitivity to erythropoietin. These mutations could be inherited or acquired.

Inherited mutations in several genes responsible for the action of erythropoietin and oxygen sensing pathways are known to cause primary congenital polycythaemia. Mutations in the *EPOR* or erythropoietin receptor gene is a well-recognised cause of primary familial and congenital polycythaemia. In addition, mutations of the genes coding for proteins in the oxygen sensing pathway cause congenital polycythaemia. These genes are *VHL, EGLN1* and *EPAS1,* which respectively code for von Hippel-Lindau, prolyl hydroxylase domain-containing protein 2 and hypoxia-inducible factor 2 alpha proteins. Some mutations of the genes coding for α- and β-globin subunits of haemoglobin are associated with an increased affinity of haemoglobin for oxygen causing tissue hypoxia leading to erythrocytosis. Also, a mutation in the *BPGM* gene results in a deficiency of 2,3-bisphosphoglycerate. Reduced 2,3-bisphosphoglycerate can increase the oxygen affinity of haemoglobin and result in tissue hypoxia. Finally, congenital methemoglobinemia resulting from an autosomal recessive deficiency of cytochrome b5 reductase cause polycythaemia.

Polycythaemia vera is the primary acquired cause of polycythaemia. It is a neoplasm that arises as a haematopoietic stem cell (HSC) disorder with a gain of function mutation in *JAK2*. Polycythaemia vera is considered as pan myelopathy which could manifest as isolated erythrocytosis, leucocytosis, thrombocytosis or any combination with associated splenomegaly or myelofibrosis.

Table 16.1. Aetiology of polycythaemia

Absolute Polycythaemia
Primary polycythaemia
Primary polycythaemia due to inherited genetic mutations
Mutations in erythropoietin receptor gene (*EPOR)*
Mutations in genes coding for proteins in the oxygen sensing pathway (*VHL, EGLN1* and *EPAS1)*
High oxygen affinity haemoglobin
Deficiency of 2,3-bisphosphoglycerate (*BPGM* mutations)
Congenital methemoglobinemia
Primary polycythaemia due to inherited genetic mutations
Polycythaemia vera (*JAK2* mutation)
Secondary polycythaemia
Tissue hypoxia-related
Chronic lung disease
Cyanotic congenital heart diseases
Carbon monoxide poisoning
High altitude
Sleep apnoea
Obesity hypoventilation syndrome
Local renal hypoxia-related
Renal artery stenosis
Renal cysts
Hydronephrosis
Erythropoietin secreting tumours
Hemangioblastoma
Meningioma
Hepatocellular carcinoma
Pheochromocytoma
Renal cell carcinoma
Relative Polycythaemia
Acute dehydration
Burns
Plasma leakage
Diuretic use

Secondary polycythaemia occurs as a result of excessive production of erythropoietin or excessive activation of the erythropoietin pathway. Most often it is due to the physiological response to tissue hypoxia but can also occur from autonomous erythropoietin production due to erythropoietin-secreting tumours. Polycythaemia in response to hypoxia is caused by chronic lung disease, cyanotic congenital heart diseases, carbon monoxide poisoning, high altitude and hypoventilation syndromes including sleep apnoea. Local renal hypoxia due to renal artery stenosis, renal cysts and hydronephrosis cause increased erythropoietin secretion and secondary polycythaemia. Some tumours such as hemangioblastoma, meningioma, hepatocellular carcinoma, pheochromocytoma and renal cell carcinoma cause autonomous production of erythropoietin, causing secondary polycythaemia.

Clinical Manifestations

Symptoms of polycythaemia are related to hyperviscosity, thrombosis or bleeding. Hyperviscosity could result in symptoms like chest pain, abdominal pain, myalgia, weakness, fatigue, blurred vision, headache, paraesthesia, transient loss of vision and slow mentation. Polycythaemia is a thrombophilic condition that causes arterial or venous thrombosis in unusual sites. Venous thrombosis occurs in mesenteric, hepatic, portal or retinal veins while arterial thrombosis can manifest as digital infarcts and ischemic strokes. Bleeding in children with polycythaemia usually presents as epistaxis or gastrointestinal bleeding. Cyanosis can be present in chronic hypoxic conditions associated with polycythaemia. Plethoric facies is also a common clinical sign of polycythaemia.

Unexplained fever, excessive sweating, weight loss, pruritus and erythromyelgia are symptoms associated with polycythaemia vera. Hepatosplenomegaly is a recognised physical sign of polycythaemia vera, and abdominal masses may present in conditions with erythropoietin secreting tumours. Approximately 5% of individuals with polycythaemia vera develop malignant transformation particularly to acute myeloid leukaemia which is often refractory to treatment.

Investigations

Polycythaemia is usually found as an incidental finding when evaluating for a different clinical concern. A full blood count is helpful in confirming the diagnosis as well as to reveal abnormalities related to leucocytes and platelets. A peripheral blood film may provide clues for the diagnosis; leucoerythroblastic blood picture may suggest myeloproliferative neoplasm. Serum erythropoietin level is used to differentiate primary from secondary polycythaemia. Elevated erythropoietin is associated with secondary polycythaemia. Low serum ferritin and low folate levels are commonly associated with primary polycythaemia. Abnormal renal functions and liver functions are associated with secondary polycythaemia.

Testing for *JAK2* mutation is not recommended in all patients. It is analysed if the individual has clinical features of polycythaemia vera or if erythropoietin is low. The presence of *JAK2* mutation is not pathognomonic, and the same mutation is present in essential thrombocytosis and primary myelofibrosis, but erythrocytosis only manifests in polycythaemia vera. However, when an individual present with erythrocytosis, leucocytosis and thrombocytosis with or without splenomegaly, the diagnosis of polycythaemia vera can be established regardless of mutation analysis.

Treatment

Mild polycythaemia does not require treatment. Treatment is indicated to children with haematocrit >65-70% to alleviate symptoms of hyperviscosity and to decrease the risk of thrombosis. These patients should be treated with periodic phlebotomy. Patients with polycythaemia could have concomitant iron deficiency due to the high demand for iron due to increased RBC production. Iron deficiency causes microcytosis, and microcytic RBCs are more rigid, therefore increases the risk of thrombosis.

Regular assessment of iron status and treatment of iron deficiency is important in children with polycythaemia.

The mainstay of treatment of polycythaemia vera is periodic phlebotomy to decrease haematocrit. In addition, low-dose aspirin is recommended for patients with thrombocytosis to prevent thrombosis and to relieve microvascular symptoms. Patients with high-risk polycythaemia vera require cytoreductive therapy with hydroxyurea, interferon-α or busulfan. Ruxolitinib is used in individuals who are unresponsive to hydroxyurea.

Prognosis

Prognosis of patients with polycythaemia depends on the cause. The median survival of patients with polycythaemia vera is approximately 14 years. Leucocytosis, venous thrombosis and leucoerythroblastic blood picture are recognised as poor prognostic factors, whereas thrombocytosis and pruritus are considered as better prognostic factors.

References

Bento, C. 2018. "Genetic basis of congenital erythrocytosis." *Int J Lab Hematol* 40 Suppl 1:62-67. doi: 10.1111/ijlh.12828.

Lee, G., and M. O. Arcasoy. 2015. "The clinical and laboratory evaluation of the patient with erythrocytosis." *Eur J Intern Med* 26 (5):297-302. doi: 10.1016/j.ejim.2015.03.007.

McMullin, M. F. 2016a. "Congenital erythrocytosis." *Int J Lab Hematol* 38 Suppl 1:59-65. doi: 10.1111/ijlh.12506.

McMullin, M. F. 2016b. "Investigation and Management of Erythrocytosis." *Curr Hematol Malig Rep* 11 (5):342-7. doi: 10.1007/s11899-016-0334-1.

McMullin, M. F. F., A. J. Mead, S. Ali, C. Cargo, F. Chen, J. Ewing, M. Garg, A. Godfrey, S. Knapper, D. P. McLornan, J. Nangalia, M. Sekhar, F. Wadelin, and C. N. Harrison. 2019. "A guideline for the management of specific situations in polycythaemia vera and secondary erythrocytosis: A British Society for Haematology Guideline." *Br J Haematol* 184 (2):161-175. doi: 10.1111/bjh.15647.

Mimouni, F. B., P. Merlob, S. Dollberg, and D. Mandel. 2011. "Neonatal polycythaemia: critical review and a consensus statement of the Israeli Neonatology Association." *Acta Paediatr* 100 (10):1290-6. doi: 10.1111/j.1651-2227.2011.02305.x.

Pillai, A. A., S. Fazal, and H. M. Babiker. 2020. "Polycythemia." In *StatPearls*. Treasure Island (FL): StatPearls Publishing Copyright © 2020, StatPearls Publishing LLC.

Spivak, J. L. 2019. "How I treat polycythemia vera." *Blood* 134 (4):341-352. doi: 10.1182/blood.2018834044.

Chapter 17

NEONATAL POLYCYTHAEMIA

Tharindi Suriapperuma and Sachith Mettananda*

Department of Paediatrics, University of Kelaniya, Ragama, Sri Lanka

Newborn babies have higher haemoglobin and haematocrit compared to infants and older children. Neonatal polycythaemia is characterised by significantly higher venous haematocrit compared to normal values for the gestational and postnatal age. Many neonates with polycythaemia are asymptomatic and are detected incidentally. Approximately 1-2% of newborns born at sea level and nearly 5% born at high altitude have polycythaemia.

DEFINITION

Haemoglobin concentration more than two standard deviations above the mean for gestational and postnatal age is defined as polycythaemia. In

* Corresponding Author's Email: sachith.mettananda@kln.ac.lk.

term neonates, polycythaemia is diagnosed when the peripheral venous haematocrit is >65% or haemoglobin is >22g/dL.

There are several factors that influence the haematocrit of neonates. These include gestational age, degree of placental transfusion and site and timing of blood sampling. Blood taken from capillaries has a higher haematocrit compared to venous blood. Haematocrit of a healthy neonate reaches a peak at two hours after birth and gradually decrease over the next 12-18 hours.

Pathophysiology

Clinical manifestations and effects of polycythaemia are due to hyperviscosity, reduced organ perfusion and increased erythrocyte break down. The volume status of the neonate, whether hypervolaemia or hypovolaemia, contributes to the clinical manifestations. Hyperviscosity may result in decreased cerebral blood flow. However, some studies suggest that reduced cerebral perfusion in polycythaemia could be due to a vascular response.

Aetiology

Neonatal polycythaemia occurs either due to increased erythropoiesis or increased erythrocyte transfusion. Causes of polycythaemia can be classified according to the volume status of the neonate into normovolaemic, hypervolaemic or hypovolaemic polycythaemia.

Normal intravascular volume with increased RBC mass is referred to as normovolaemic polycythaemia. Chronic intrauterine hypoxia is the leading cause of normovolaemic polycythaemia. Placental insufficiency and several maternal conditions such as preeclampsia, chronic hypertension, vascular disorders and cardiac or pulmonary disease cause intrauterine hypoxia. Maternal diabetes, maternal smoking, high altitude and propranolol use in mothers also contribute to neonatal polycythaemia. In addition, large for gestational age babies and neonates with congenital adrenal hyperplasia, hypothyroidism, hyperthyroidism or chromosomal abnormalities (trisomy 13, 18 or 21) are prone to develop polycythaemia due to increased erythropoiesis. Also, polycythaemia may occur in neonates born post-term compared to term or preterm neonates.

In hypervolaemic polycythaemia, both intravascular volume and RBC mass are increased. Twin-twin transfusion and maternal-fetal transfusion are two occasions where a newborn is receiving passive transfusions. Delayed cord clamping allows the transfer of extra blood to the newborn, causing polycythaemia. In hypovolaemic polycythaemia, there is a relative increase in RBC mass to plasma volume. This commonly occurs following dehydration.

Clinical Manifestations

Most neonates with polycythaemia are asymptomatic. In symptomatic neonates, symptoms generally appear within the first 48-72 hours. The most commonly reported symptoms are poor feeding, vomiting, lethargy, jitteriness, apnoea and cyanosis. Hypoglycaemia, hyperbilirubinaemia and necrotising enterocolitis are frequently associated complications of neonatal polycythaemia. Hypoglycaemia is most probably due to increased utilisation of glucose by increased RBC mass. Other clinical features that have an uncertain association to neonatal polycythaemia are respiratory distress, tachycardia, irritability, haematuria, renal vein thrombosis, priapism, gallstones, increased pulmonary vascular resistance and seizures. Neonatal polycythaemia can also lead to behavioural issues, developmental delay and specific learning disabilities in childhood.

Investigations and Diagnosis

Haematocrit is not routinely measured in all newborns. When polycythaemia is suspected, a screening capillary haematocrit is performed. If capillary blood haematocrit is above 65%, neonatal polycythaemia should be confirmed by performing a venous haematocrit.

Treatment

Management of neonatal polycythaemia depends on the haematocrit and symptoms of the neonate. Asymptomatic neonates with a haematocrit of 65-70% should be carefully observed with repeat haematocrit in 12-24 hours. These neonates should be adequately hydrated and monitored for hypoglycaemia and hyperbilirubinaemia. Asymptomatic neonates with a haematocrit of 70-75% could still be observed as above without intervention. However, some centres would prefer to initiate intravenous fluid in these neonates.

All symptomatic neonates with haematocrit >65% and asymptomatic neonates with haematocrit >75% require intervention to control polycythaemia. Partial exchange transfusion by removing blood from an umbilical venous catheter and replacing 0.9% sodium chloride into a peripheral vein is the preferred intervention. The exchange blood volume is calculated targeting a desired haematocrit (Hct) of 55%.

$$\text{Exchange volume} = [(\text{observed Hct} - \text{desired Hct}) \times \text{blood volume}] \div \text{observed Hct}$$

Partial exchange transfusion helps to reduce the haematocrit but does not affect the long-term outcome of polycythaemia. Increased risk of necrotising enterocolitis had been observed following partial exchange transfusion for polycythaemia.

Prognosis

Long term prognosis of neonatal polycythaemia or its treatment is uncertain. The available evidence suggests the long-term clinical outcome depends on the complications and other associated factors such as hypoglycaemia and placental insufficiency rather than polycythaemia itself.

References

Bashir, B. A., and S. A. Othman. 2019. "Neonatal polycythaemia." *Sudan J Paediatr* 19 (2):81-83. doi: 10.24911/sjp.106-1566075225.

McMullin, M. F. 2016. "Congenital erythrocytosis." *Int J Lab Hematol* 38 Suppl 1:59-65. doi: 10.1111/ijlh.12506.

Mimouni, F. B., P. Merlob, S. Dollberg, and D. Mandel. 2011. "Neonatal polycythaemia: critical review and a consensus statement of the Israeli Neonatology Association." *Acta Paediatr* 100 (10):1290-6. doi: 10. 1111/j.1651-2227.2011.02305.x.

ABOUT THE AUTHORS

Prof Sachith Mettananda
Professor in Paediatrics and Consultant Paediatrician
Department of Paediatrics, Faculty of Medicine, University of Kelaniya,
Ragama, Sri Lanka

Professor Sachith Mettananda, MBBS(Col), MD-Paediatrics(Col), DPhil(Oxon) and FRCP(Edin) is currently a Professor in Paediatrics and the Head of the Department of Paediatrics at University of Kelaniya and a Consultant Paediatrician at the Colombo North Teaching Hospital, Ragama, Sri Lanka. He has authored many book chapters and numerous research publications on paediatric red blood cell disorders of which many are in high impact journals including *Blood, Nature Communications, Haematologica, British Journal of Haematology, Hematology/ Oncology Clinics of North America, Scientific Reports, Paediatric Blood and Cancer* and *Experimental Hematology*. He has received many national and international awards including Commonwealth Scholarship Award by the British Government (2012), President's Award for scientific publications by the Sri Lankan Government (2011, 2015 and 2016) and Ten Outstanding Young Persons in Sri Lanka Award (2016). He has over fifteen years of experience in treating patients with paediatric red blood cell disorders and teaching medical undergraduates and postgraduate trainees in paediatrics. He has also served in the capacity of a council member of the Sri Lanka College of Paediatricians (2016-2018), founder secretary of the Rare Disease Forum of Sri Lanka (2017-2019) and a member of the National Thalassaemia Council (2016-todate) and National Health Research Council of Sri Lanka (2017-todate).

Dr Duantida Songdej

Assistant Professor in Paediatrics and Consultant Paediatric Haematologist
Department of Paediatrics, Faculty of Medicine Ramathibodi Hospital,
Mahidol University, Bangkok, Thailand

Dr Duantida Songdej is a medical graduate with first class honours from Faculty of Medicine Ramathibodi Hospital, Mahidol University, Bangkok, Thailand, where she also did her paediatric residency and paediatric haematology and oncology fellowship training. Dr Songdej completed her Doctor of Philosophy (DPhil) degree in the Higgs Laboratory of the Molecular Haematology Unit, Weatherall Institute of Molecular Medicine, University of Oxford, United Kingdom. During her DPhil training, she initiated the international registry of survivors with Haemoglobin Bart's hydrops fetalis syndrome, the result of which was recently published in *Blood* and the project is on-going. Currently, Dr Songdej is an Assistant Professor in Paediatrics and is a consultant in Hematology-Oncology Unit, Department of Paediatrics, Faculty of Medicine Ramathibodi Hospital, Mahidol University. Her work and research mainly involve patients with red blood cell disorders. She leads haematology and thalassemia clinic and sets up a variety of molecular methods for diagnosis of rare inherited haemolytic anaemias. Dr Songdej is also a member of the Thai national subcommittee on red blood cell disorders of the Thai Society of Haematology. She was an invited speaker nationally and internationally during the past 3-4 years and she has authored over 25 publications.

Dr Tharindi Suriapperuma
Lecturer in Paediatrics
Department of Paediatrics, Faculty of Medicine, University of Kelaniya, Sri Lanka

Dr Tharindi Suriapperuma, MBBS, DCH(Col) and MD-Paediatrics(Col) is currently a lecturer of the Department of Paediatrics at Faculty of Medicine, University of Kelaniya and a senior registrar in general paediatrics at Colombo North Teaching Hospital, Ragama, Sri Lanka. She graduated MBBS with second (upper) class honours from the University of Kelaniya winning three distinctions, gold medals for Paediatrics and Surgery and the University of Kelaniya Alumni Association gold medal for the best performance at the final examination for medical degree. She obtained MD-Paediatrics from the Postgraduate Institute of Medicine, Colombo with Prof Sanath P. Lamabadusuriya gold medal for best performance in the clinical examination and Prof. Priyani E. Soysa gold medal for best overall performance. She has presented number of papers in national and international scientific meetings.

INDEX

#

A

B

F

G

H

I

J

K

L

M

N

O

P

R

S